Atlas of
Lung **Cancer**
AND OTHER CHEST TUMORS

Atlas of
Lung **Cancer**
AND OTHER CHEST TUMORS

Editors:

Professor Dame Margaret Turner-Warwick DBE DM, PhD,
DSc(Hon), FRCP(Edin.), FRACP, FACP, FFOM, PRCP
President
Royal College of Physicians
London

Dr Margaret E.Hodson MD, MSc, FRCP, DA
Reader in Respiratory Medicine
National Heart and Lung Institute
The Royal Brompton Hospital
London

Professor Bryan Corrin MD, FRCPath
Professor of Thoracic Pathology
National Heart and Lung Institute
The Royal Brompton Hospital
London

Dr Ian H.Kerr MA, MBBChir, FRCP, FRCR
Honorary Consulting Radiologist
The Royal Brompton Hospital
London

Gower Medical Publishing • London • New York

Distributed in the USA and Canada by:
J B Lippincott Company
East Washington Square
Philadelphia
PA 19105
USA

Distributed in the UK and Continental Europe by:
Gower Medical Publishing
Middlesex House
34–42 Cleveland Street
London W1P 5FB
UK

Distributed in Australia and New Zealand by:
Harper and Row (Australia) Pty Ltd
PO Box 226
Artarmon
NSW 2064
Australia

Distributed in Southeast Asia, Hong Kong, India and Pakistan by:
Harper and Row (Asia) Pte Ltd
37 Jalan Pemimpin 02–01
Singapore 2057

Distributed in Japan by:
Nankodo Co Ltd
42–6 Hongo 3-chome
Bunkyo-ku
Tokyo 113
Japan

Typesetting by M to N Typesetters, London
Text set in Bembo; captions set in Univers
Illustrations originated in Hong Kong by Imago Productions Ltd
Text origination and page make up by Hilo Offset Ltd, Colchester
Produced by Mandarin Offset
Printed in Hong Kong

Publisher:
Fiona Foley

Project Manager:
Alison Whitehouse

Design and Layout:
Tim Friers
Pete Walter Wilder

Index:
Laurence Errington

Production:
Susan Bishop

British Library Cataloguing in Publication Data:
Atlas of lung cancer and other chest tumours.
 I. Turner-Warwick, Professor Margaret
 616.2

Library of Congress Cataloging in Publication Data:
Atlas of lung cancer and other chest tumors / Dame Margaret
 Turner-Warwick ... [et al.].
 Includes index.
 1. Lungs--Tumors--Atlases. 2. Chest--Tumors--Atlases.
 3. Smoking--Health aspects. I. Turner-Warwick, Margaret, 1924–
 [DNLM: 1. Lung Neoplasms--atlases. 2. Smoking--adverse effects
 --atlases. 3. Thoracic Neoplasms--atlases. WF 17 A8805]
 RC280.L8A85   1991
 616.99'424--dc20

ISBN 0-397-44838-4

PREFACE

This Atlas aims to improve the understanding of all who are involved in the care of lung cancer patients, by using visual material. While its main theme is the radiographic presentations and their use in diagnosis, no discussion of lung cancer can omit its major cause, thus a chapter on smoking and its effects on the lungs is included. It is hoped that students and trainee and consultant physicians will find it useful: we feel that, in this field, the visual image can often convey more information than a written description.

The Atlas is not intended to be a textbook, its emphasis is on the image, and the text is only a brief summary to complement the pictures. (Readers who require further information should consult one of the excellent textbooks on respiratory medicine now available.)

We would like to thank all those who have provided material for the Atlas and we hope our acknowledgements are complete. We apologise for any omissions.

Finally we would like to thank Gower Medical Publishing for their co-operation in the publication of this Atlas.

CONTRIBUTORS TO CHAPTER 1

Dr J.G. Ayres BSc MB BS MD FRCP

Consultant Physician in Respiratory Medicine
East Birmingham Hospital

Dr P.J. Rees MD FRCP

Consultant Physician and Senior Lecturer in Medicine
United Medical and Dental School (UMDS), Guy's Hospital

CONTENTS

1 *Smoking*

J.G. Ayres and P.J. Rees

Smoking is acknowledged by all except the tobacco industry as the cause of many thousands of premature deaths and considerable morbidity from conditions such as lung cancer, chronic bronchitis and emphysema, and ischaemic heart disease. In this chapter the stress is on respiratory disease and data are given only where the evidence for cigarette smoke as a causal agent is good; animal work has been excluded. Although the weight of information is overwhelming that cigarettes cause disease, there is clearly a need for much more research, particularly in the area of mechanisms of smoking-induced damage. On the public health front the impending pandemic of smoking-induced disease in Third World countries is a major concern, an additional health load that these already stressed countries can do without.

TOBACCO CONSUMPTION

Over the period of the 1950s and 1960s the gap between the number of men and women smoking steadily narrowed (Fig. 1.1). The proportion of men who smoke has steadily declined from the early 1970s and the trend amongst women has been following a similar decline since the mid 1970s so that both rates are now below forty percent. Over the thirteen years from 1972 to 1984 the number of adult male smokers fell by nearly one-third and adult female smokers by one-fifth, however, the current rates suggest that there are still around fifteen million smokers in the United Kingdom together with ten million ex-smokers.

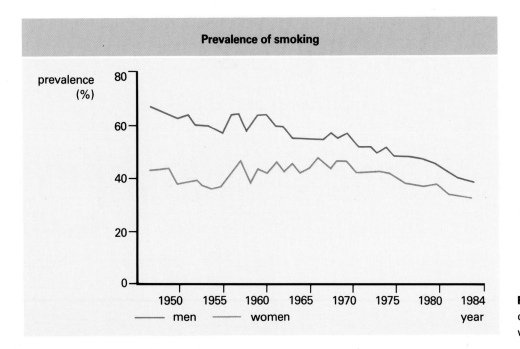

Fig. 1.1 Prevalence of current cigarette smoking in men and women in the UK from 1948 to 1984.

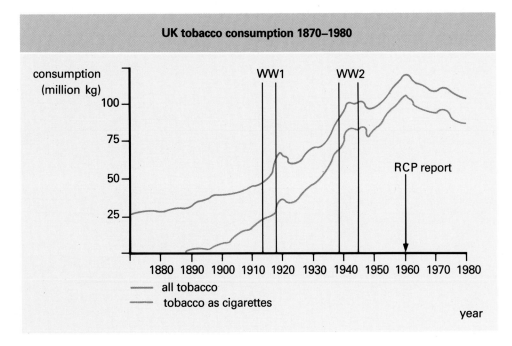

Fig. 1.2 Total tobacco consumption in the UK, 1870 to 1980. The upper line is for all tobacco, the lower for tobacco sold as cigarettes (RCP = Royal College of Physicians).

Weekly cigarette consumption 1972–1984

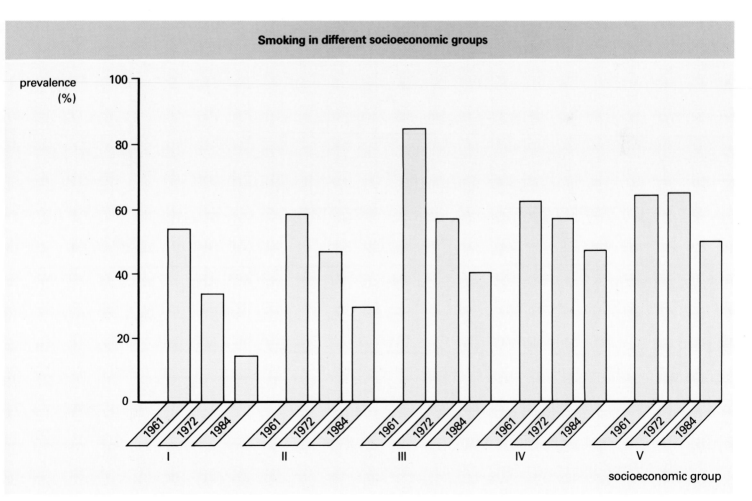

consumption

140

130

120

110

100

90

80

1972 1974 1976 1978 1980 1982 1984
year

● ● male
● ● female

Information available on the total tobacco consumption in the United Kingdom over the last 100 years (Fig. 1.2) shows a steady increase throughout the century up until the early 1960s. Both World Wars were associated with a step up in the trend. The downturn of the mid 1960s occurred in association with the report from the Royal College of Physicians on the adverse effects of smoking. The average weekly consumption per smoker began to fall later than did the overall consumption and the numbers smoking, possibly because smokers of a greater number of cigarettes found it more difficult to stop. It was not until the start of the 1980s that a downturn in average consumption per smoker was evident (Fig. 1.3). Between 1972 and 1984 sales of packeted cigarettes fell by twenty-five per-cent from 130,500 million to 99,300 million. Cigar sales are

Fig. 1.3 Average weekly cigarette consumption for male and female smokers from 1972 to 1984.

Smoking in different socioeconomic groups

prevalence (%)

100

80

60

40

20

0

1961 1972 1984   1961 1972 1984   1961 1972 1984   1961 1972 1984   1961 1972 1984

I   II   III   IV   V

socioeconomic group

Fig. 1.4 Prevalence of smoking in males of different socioeconomic classes, 1961, 1972 and 1984.

3

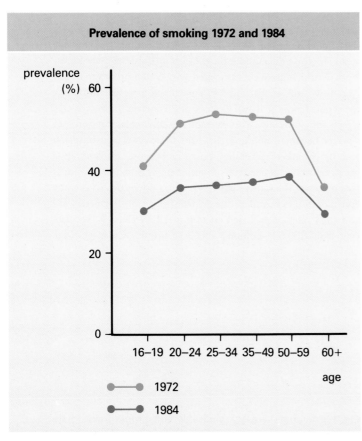

Prevalence of smoking 1972 and 1984

prevalence (%)

1972
1984

also falling, from 1730 million in 1978 to 1495 million in 1983. Differences in prevalence of smoking between different socio-economic groups have become more marked over the last 20 years so that by 1984 only seventeen percent of professional groups were smokers compared with forty-nine percent of unskilled manual workers (Fig. 1.4). The prevalence of smoking also varies with age but all age groups have managed to decrease their smoking rates over the last fifteen years (Fig. 1.5). There are some worrying statistics in the younger age groups, especially amongst girls. In the sixteen to nineteen year age group more women (thirty-two percent) than men (twenty-nine percent) smoked in 1984 and women in this age range were the only group to show an increase between 1982 and 1984. In eleven to fifteen year olds the prevalence of regular cigarette smoking fell from eleven percent in 1982 and thirteen percent in 1984 to seven percent in 1986 amongst boys, but amongst girls the prevalence remained almost constant at eleven percent in 1982, thirteen percent in 1984 and twelve percent in 1986.

Fig. 1.5 Prevalence of smoking by age in 1972 and 1984 (male and female combined data).

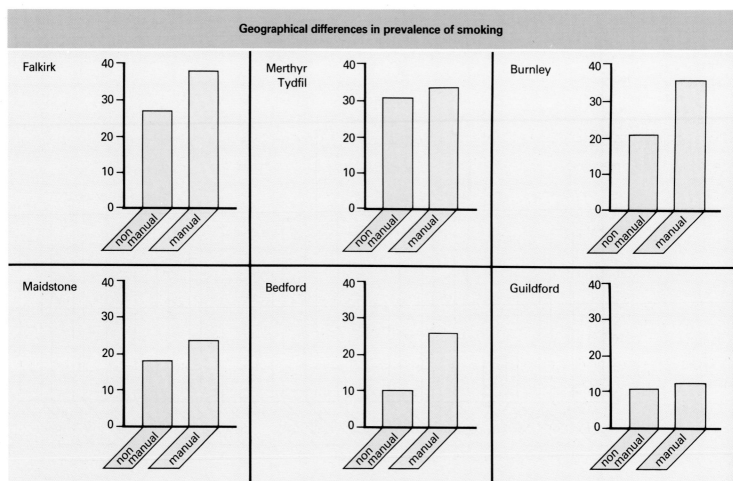

Geographical differences in prevalence of smoking

Falkirk

Merthyr Tydfil

Burnley

Maidstone

Bedford

Guildford

Fig. 1.6 Geographical differences in the prevalence of smoking 20 or more cigarettes daily among middle-aged men.

Rates vary greatly in different countries and the prevalence rates for smoking in the UK are not consistent across the country. As with many other social factors there is to some extent a North–South divide or at least a difference between the South-East and the rest of the country. This was brought out in the British Regional Heart study, some examples from which are shown in Fig. 1.6. To take extreme examples, fourteen percent of Guildford manual workers smoked compared with forty percent of a similar group in Grimsby.

We are currently seeing the damage caused by cigarette smoking over the last fifty to sixty years and Fig. 1.7 shows that of the developed countries the UK is high in the ranking of cigarette consumption over this period. The recent decline in smoking rates is encouraging but not enough to avoid a great many problems over the next thirty to forty years. Increasing rates of smoking and high tar levels in many Third World countries will ensure that this becomes a truly international problem (Fig. 1.8).

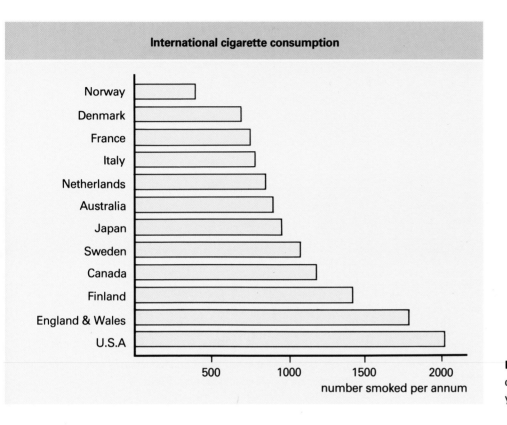

Fig. 1.7 International cigarette consumption (number smoked per year) (average values 1920–1959).

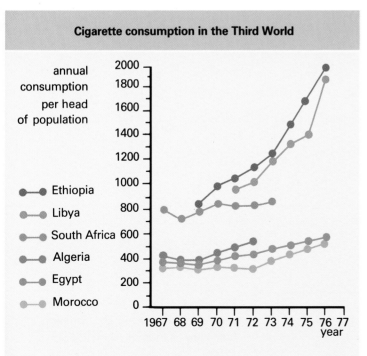

Fig. 1.8 Increasing trends of cigarette consumption in Third World countries.

MORTALITY

Cigarette smoking is associated with an increased mortality from a number of diseases comprising many of the major causes of death in the United Kingdom. Figure 1.9 shows the number of deaths caused by some of these conditions in 1984, according to figures from the Office for Population Censuses and Surveys (OPCS). Tumours of the bladder, pancreas and some other sites are also known to be associated with smoking. The Royal College of Physicians has estimated that 100,000 people in the United Kingdom every year are killed by smoking.

Figure 1.10 shows the changes which have occurred over ten years in the death rates from carcinoma of the lung and chronic bronchitis and emphysema. Mortality from all causes combined

Mortality for smoking-related diseases		
Cause	ICD codes	Mortality
Chronic bronchitis and emphysema	491, 492 496, 416	25,318
Cancer of the lung	162	35,739
Cancer of the larynx	161	779
Cancer of the oesophagus	150	4297
Ischaemic heart disease	410–414	157,506
Cerebrovascular disease	430–438	71,470

Fig. 1.9 Mortality (absolute numbers) for diseases associated with smoking (England and Wales, 1984).

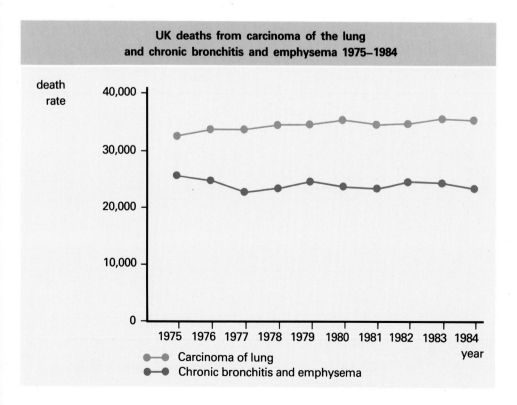

Fig. 1.10 Annual UK death rate from carcinoma of the lung and chronic bronchitis and emphysema (1975–1986).

increases with the amount smoked. This is usually expressed as a mortality ratio as shown in Fig. 1.11. The mortality rate for non-smokers is shown as unity and all the other groups are then compared to this. This data is taken from a number of different sources and it can be seen that the ratio increases steadily with consumption. Ex-smokers have an intermediate mortality rate, but they are a difficult group to cope with in such statistics since some of them may have given up smoking because of relevant symptoms. The risks increase with the length of history of smoking. Figure 1.12 shows mortality ratios for males aged forty-five to fifty-four years according to the age at which they started to smoke.

The mortality ratios become even more striking when they are calculated for individual smoking-related conditions rather

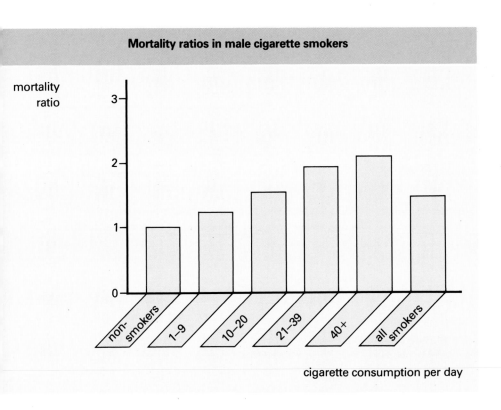

Fig. 1.11 Standardized mortality ratios in male cigarette smokers according to the number of smoked. cigarettes

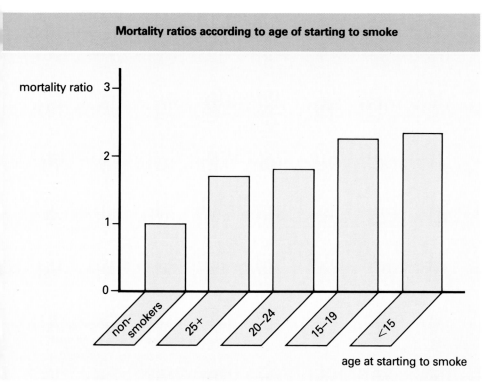

Fig. 1.12 Mortality ratios for male cigarette smokers (aged 45–64) according to age of starting to smoke.

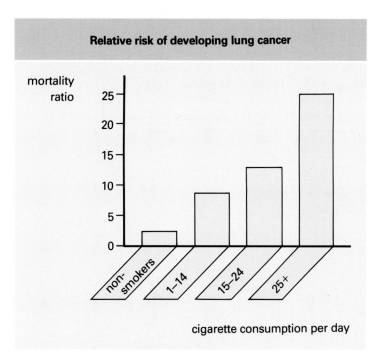

Fig. 1.13 Relative risk of developing lung cancer for male smokers according to cigarette consumption.

Fig. 1.14 Mortality rates for chronic bronchitis and emphysema in males according to tobacco consumption.

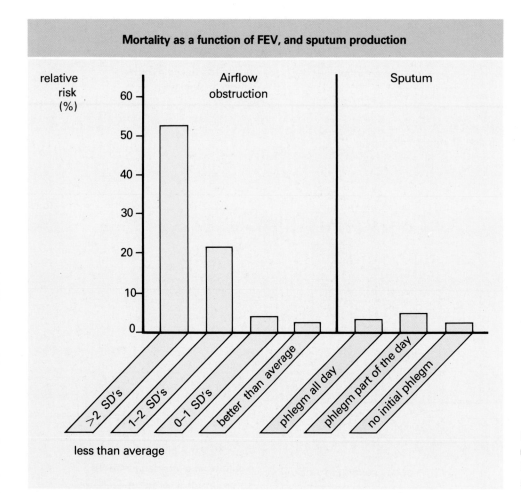

Fig. 1.15 Mortality expressed as relative risk of dying as a function of initial lung function (FEV$_1$/ht^3) and of sputum production.

than overall mortality. Doll and Peto showed that smokers of over 25 cigarettes daily had a risk of carcinoma of the bronchus over 25 times that of non-smokers (Fig. 1.13), and similar findings are seen for chronic bronchitis and emphysema (Fig. 1.14).

MORBIDITY

Morbidity can be defined as the non-fatal health load to a community or, on an individual basis, as the economic and social effects of the symptoms and non-fatal consequences of a specific condition.

Although we confine ourselves here to morbidity with respect to the respiratory tract, it is clear that morbidity from cigarette smoking-induced, non-respiratory diseases such as ischaemic heart disease, peripheral vascular disease, peptic ulcer and carcinomas of the bladder and oesophagus is high, although difficult to quantitate epidemiologically.

We do not consider in any detail carcinomas of the naso-pharynx, larynx and bronchus. Morbidity from malignancies is admittedly high, not only from symptoms, notably dyspnoea and pain, but also from the effects of chemo- and radiotherapy. In terms of health load such treatment and community care is also expensive. One also has to consider the psychological load both to the patient and to their relatives and friends. Neverthe-

less, the main morbidity due to the effects of smoking on the respiratory tract is related to diseases of the airways, causing cough with sputum production and airflow obstruction.

The morbidity due to chronic bronchitis can be measured in terms of hospital admissions, time lost from work and consultations to general practitioners. Between 1971 and 1981 the prevalence of chronic bronchitis in general practice fell by about half for both men and women. Although time lost from work can no longer be used for accurate assessment of morbidity since the advent of self-certification in the UK, an approximate figure of 50 million working days lost per annum is likely to be a reasonable estimate. Cigarette smoking causes both airflow obstruction and mucus hypersecretion but these seem to develop independently of each other, as subsequent mortality relates to the degree of airflow obstruction, not mucus hypersecretion (Fig. 1.15).

COUGH

The MRC definition of chronic bronchitis concerns sputum production rather than airflow obstruction. Classically the term is applied to patients coughing up sputum on at least three consecutive months for more than two successive years. Sputum comprises the combined secretions of the bronchial mucus glands and the goblet cells, both of which show an

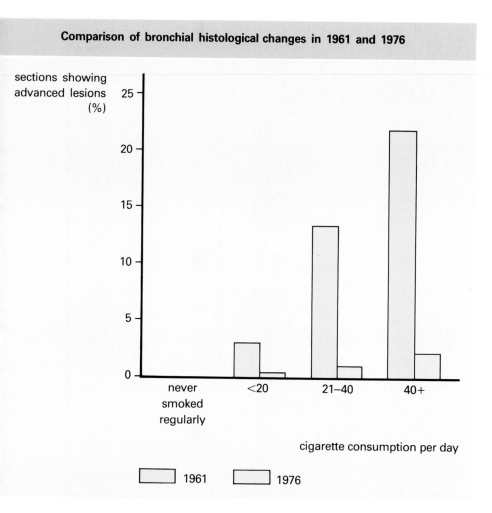

Comparison of bronchial histological changes in 1961 and 1976

cigarette consumption per day

1961   1976

Fig. 1.16 Change in bronchial histological changes from 1961 to 1976 according to cigarette consumption.

increase in size and number in chronic bronchitis. Auerbach assessed certain histological changes — loss of cilia, cells with atypia, basal cell hyperplasia — and showed that these histological changes have become less marked over the years (Fig. 1.16), although the dose–response effect of cigarette consumption is still maintained. There is a clear relationship between sputum production and smoking (Fig. 1.17) for both males and females. Stopping smoking can result in reversal of mucus hypersecretion, but in ex-smokers who continue to produce sputum, the inflammatory process continues to involve both central and peripheral airways. This more widespread effect of smoking in certain individuals will be associated with a compounding factor such as airborne pollution. A study of British postal workers showed that persistent respiratory symptoms were more common in urban smokers than in rural smokers (Fig. 1.18) controlling for social class. This difference becomes more noticeable with increasing cigarette consumption.

Smokers not only produce more sputum but also have impaired mucociliary clearance. This is partly caused by loss of cilia associated with areas of squamous metaplasia but is also related to dysfunction of the remaining cilia, either overwhelmed by the increased volume of secretions being produced

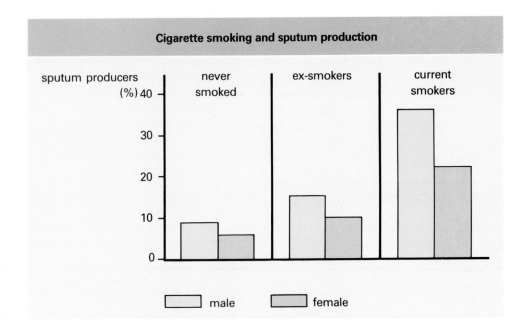

Fig. 1.17 Association of cigarette smoking with sputum production.

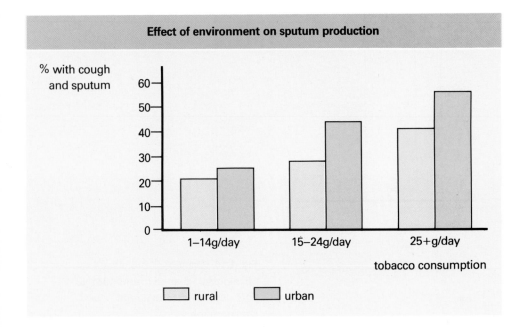

Fig. 1.18 Compounding effect of cigarette smoking and an urban environment on cough with sputum production.

or inhibited functionally by the gas phase of cigarette smoke (Fig. 1.19). Radionuclide studies in symptomless cigarette smokers have shown that mucociliary clearance is impaired compared to non-smokers, with a significantly prolonged residence time.

AIRFLOW OBSTRUCTION

It has been proposed that changes in lung function (FEV_1) with time in smokers would follow certain pathways: some smokers would show a slow deterioration in lung function with age similar to that seen in non-smokers, whereas others would show a rapid fall. Should these latter subjects stop smoking then their subsequent fall in lung function would progress at the same rate as non-smokers or the non-susceptible smokers. The possible effect of bronchial hyper-responsiveness in the development of chronic airflow obstruction is discussed later, but the two theories can be combined (Fig. 1.20).

Other studies have shown that the effects of cigarette smoking can be seen earlier with more sophisticated tests in subjects who are both asymptomatic and who have normal dynamic

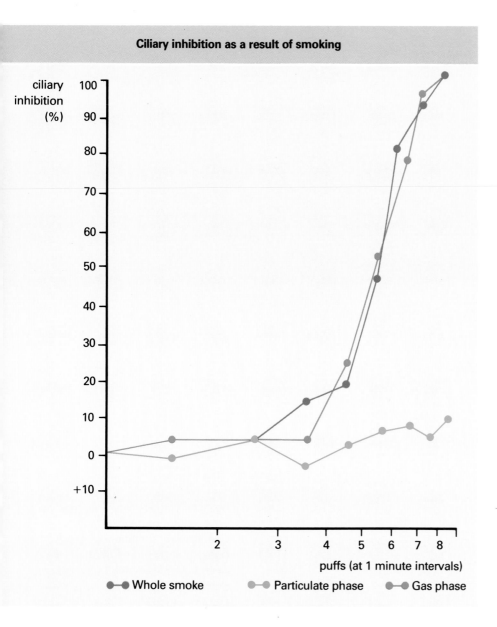

Fig. 1.19 Ciliary inhibition by the gas phase of cigarette smoke.

lung volumes. For instance, it has been shown that these subjects have abnormal nitrogen washout (Fig. 1.21) suggesting small airways involvement at an early stage in their smoking 'life' but such changes are reversible with cessation of smoking.

Smoking has been shown to be associated with an increased risk of spontaneous pneumothorax in a dose-dependent manner (Fig. 1.22).

PASSIVE SMOKING

Apart from the fact that cigarette smoke is aesthetically unpleasant to non-smokers, there is now considerable evidence that cigarette smoke inhaled passively can cause increased respiratory symptoms, airway obstruction and lung cancer.

In some smoky rooms, individuals show a reduction in attentiveness and cognitive function which is related to ambient CO levels.

Children of parents who smoke have been shown to be shorter than children not passively exposed to cigarette smoke,

even allowing for factors such as social class and low birth rate.

Exercise tolerance is reduced in patients with IHD passively exposed to cigarette smoke because of a lowered angina threshold related to ambient CO levels.

Exercise tolerance is reduced in a similar fashion in patients with chronic airflow obstruction.

The children of parents who smoke have been shown in many studies to suffer an increased incidence of respiratory symptoms and of attacks of bronchitis and pneumonia. The effect is greater when both parents smoke.

The rate of increase of FEV_1 during adolescence is reduced by up to ten percent in subjects whose mothers smoke cigarettes.

Passive smokers show reduced mid-expiratory flows (FEF 25–75) (Fig. 1.23) and flows at low lung volumes are significantly lower than predicted. The changes are similar to smokers who claim not to inhale and to smokers of up to ten cigarettes a day for more than twenty years.

Passively inhaled cigarette smoke acts as a trigger for exacerbation of asthma.

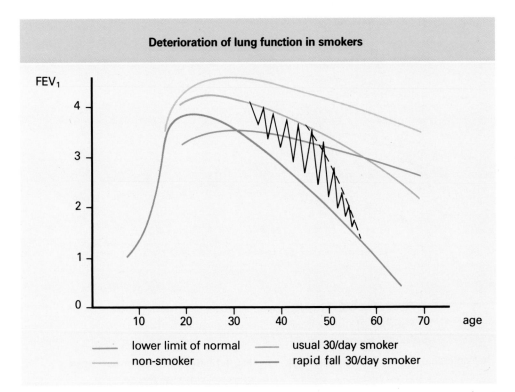

Deterioration of lung function in smokers

FEV_1

— lower limit of normal — usual 30/day smoker
— non-smoker — rapid fall 30/day smoker

Fig. 1.20 The 'Fletcher Diagram' of patterns of lung function deterioration in chronic cigarette smokers as modified by Busse to incorporate patients with a reversible element to their airflow obstruction as represented by the zig-zag decline.

Lung function changes in asymptomatic smokers

percentage abnormal

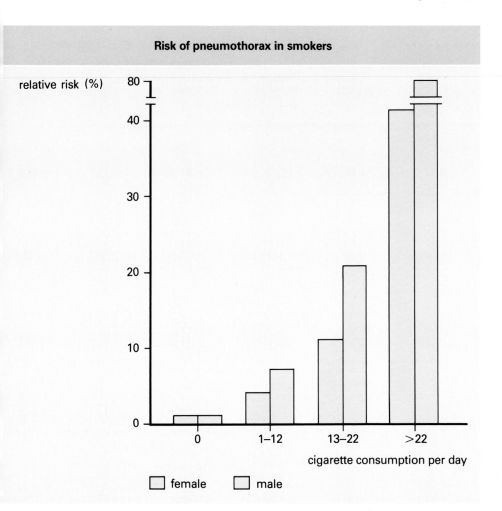

FEV₁ FVC FEV₁/FVC MMFR ΔN₂/1 CV/VC
×100

lung function parameters

☐ male smokers   ☐ female smokers

Fig. 1.21 Lung function changes in asymptomatic smokers, showing markedly reduced nitrogen washout.

Risk of pneumothorax in smokers

relative risk (%)

cigarette consumption per day

0   1–12   13–22   >22

☐ female   ☐ male

Fig. 1.22 Increased risk of pneumothorax according to cigarette consumption.

CARCINOGENESIS

In 1981 a large long term follow up study showed that non-smoking wives of cigarette-smoking Japanese men showed an increased risk of lung cancer in a dose–response manner according to the amount smoked by the husband (Fig. 1.24).

A similar finding was shown later in that year using a case control study of 59 non-smoking women who developed lung cancer. Twenty-nine cases of lung cancer were found compared to an expected number of twelve. Again a dose–response effect was shown. A meta-analysis of all published work in this area confirmed that passive smoking did increase the risk of deve-

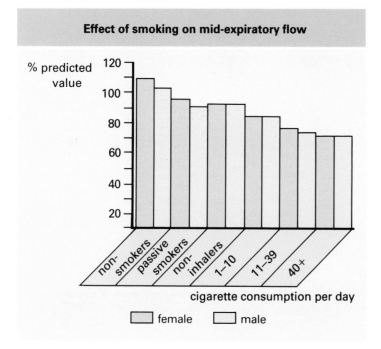

Fig. 1.23 Reduction in mid-expiratory flows in passive smokers and in active smokers, showing a dose-dependent reduction.

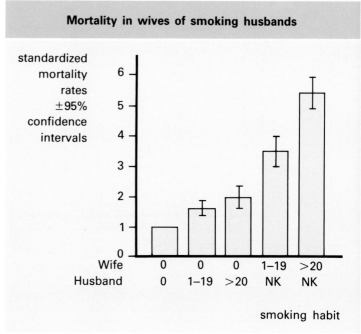

Fig. 1.24 Standardized mortality rates (+/− 95% confidence intervals) for lung cancer in wives of husbands who smoke, showing increased risk in the passive smoker.

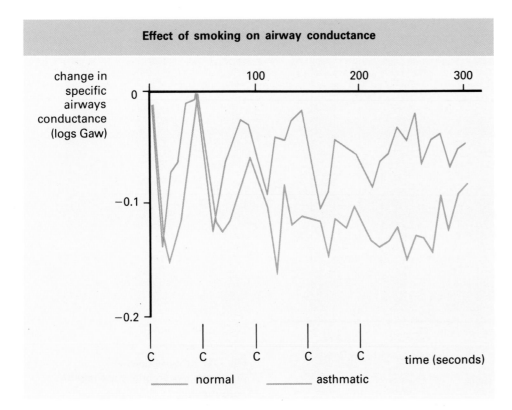

Fig. 1.25 Acute reduction in specific airways conductance with 5 puffs of cigarette smoke at 50 second intervals in normal and asthmatic subjects.

loping lung cancer in a non-smoker with an adjusted relative risk of 1.53 (i.e. fifty-three percent increased risk). On this basis about a quarter of all non-smoking lung cancers in non-smokers can be attributed to passive smoking.

MECHANISMS

Cigarette smoke is an irritant substance affecting the eyes and the respiratory tract. When measurements are made some minutes after cigarette smoking a minority of individuals, both smokers and non-smokers, show evidence of induced bronchoconstriction. However, when measurements are made after each puff of smoke from the cigarette, acute temporary changes are seen on each occasion and some subjects maintain these changes for longer (Fig. 1.25).

Although the role of inhaled cigarette smoke and probably environmental pollution is accepted in the development of chronic airflow obstruction, it is possible that chronic airflow obstruction only develops on the background of bronchial hyper-responsiveness (BHR). This hypothesis would accommodate the patient with 'asthmatic bronchitis' (Fig. 1.20), and would explain, to some extent, the group of smokers whose airways remain resistant to the effects of cigarette smoke,

comprising perhaps eighty percent of all smokers. However, although many do so, not all asthmatics who continue to smoke go on to develop an irreversible element to their airflow obstruction.

Cigarette smoke is an inflammatory agent. It recruits alveolar macrophages which attract neutrophils by means of neutrophil chemotactic factor release. Proteases are then produced with their destructive effects on collagen, elastin and fibronectins. In normal subjects there are natural inhibitors of the various proteases: α_1-protease inhibitor, procollagenase, TIMP, plasminogen activator inhibitor.

The best understood of these balancing systems is that of α_1-protease inhibitor (previously known as α_1-antitrypsin). In individuals with α_1-protease inhibitor deficiency who smoke, symptoms from chronic airflow obstruction occur fifteen to twenty years earlier than in similarly affected individuals who do not smoke. Cigarette smoke is an inhibitor of α_1-protease inhibitor so that individuals already having low levels can suffer the effects of the initially unopposed action of tissue proteases associated with day-to-day infections or inhalation of environmental toxins etc.

The alveolar macrophage (Fig. 1.26) is, therefore, fundamental in the pathogenesis of cigarette smoking induced lung damage. However, although increased numbers of macro-

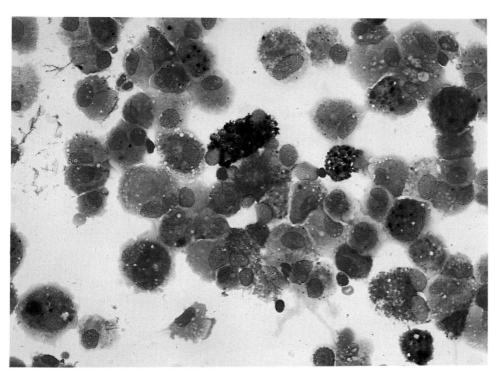

Fig. 1.26 Alveolar macrophages from a smoker.

phages are seen in the alveolar walls of smokers, in smokers who have developed emphysema the numbers show no further increase, suggesting that additional other factors are important in the pathogenesis of emphysema.

When measurements of the permeability of the lung epithelium were made after inhalation of DTPA labelled with Technetium-99m it was found that smokers had an abnormally fast clearance of the isotope from the lung (Fig. 1.27). This indicated an increased permeability of the epithelium. Studies performed in smokers who stopped smoking showed that a large part of this abnormally increased permeability was reversed within a week or two of stopping smoking. This effect is presumably related to some form of damage by the cigarette smoke but the mechanism and the implications of these findings are still unknown.

A great number of carcinogenic agents, tumour promoters and co-carcinogens have been described in tobacco smoke; these are listed in Fig. 1.28 and there are other unknown or uncharacterized substances to be added to this list.

INTERVENTION

Stopping
Several studies have shown the reduction in the relative risk of cigarette smoking related diseases and the reduction in overall

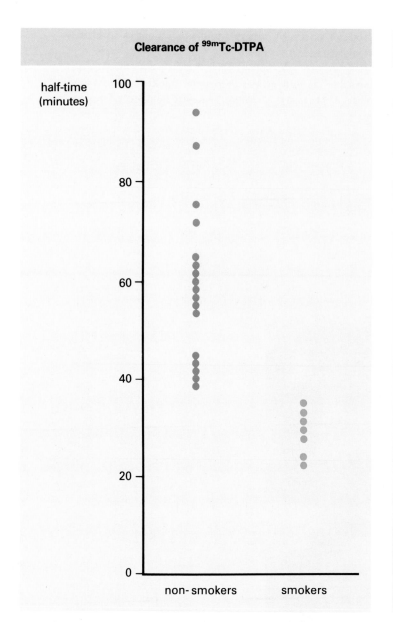

Clearance of ^{99m}Tc-DTPA

half-time (minutes)

non-smokers   smokers

Carcinogens in tobacco smoke	
Compound	**Amount in one cigarette**
Tumour initiators	
benzo(a)pyrene	10–50ng
5-methylchrysene	0.6ng
dibenz(a,h)anthracene	40ng
benzo(b)fluoranthene	30ng
benzo(j)fluoranthene	60ng
dibenzo(a,h)pyrene	present
dibenzo(a,i)pyrene	present
dibenz(a,j)acridine	3–10ng
indeno(1,2,3-cd)pyrene	4ng
benz(a)anthracene	40–70ng
chrysene	40–60ng
methylchrysenes	18ng
methylfluoranthenes	50ng
dibenz(a,c)anthracenes	present
dibenz(a,h)acridine	0.1ng
dibenzo(c,g)carbazole	0.7ng
benzo(c)phenanthrene	present
Specific lung carcinogens	
polonium-210	0.03–1.3pCi
nickel compounds	0–600ng
cadmium compounds	9–70ng
Tumour promoters	
volatile phenols	150–500µg
Co-carcinogens	
pyrene	50–200ng
methylpyrenes	30–300ng
fluoranthene	100–260ng
methylfluoranthene	180ng
benzo(g,h,i)perylene	60ng
benzo(e)pyrene	30ng
napthelenes	0.3–6.3µg
1-methylindoles	0.83µg
9-methylcarbazoles	0.14µg
4,4'-dichlorostilbene	1.5µg
catechol	200–500µg
4-alkylcatechol	10µg

Fig. 1.27 Half time of clearance (minutes) of ^{99m}Tc-DTPA in smokers and non-smokers.

Fig. 1.28 Carcinogenic agents, tumour promoters, and co-carcinogens in the particulate phase of tobacco smoke.

mortality on stopping smoking. This was originally shown by Doll and Peto in the British Doctors Study, but more recent data for carcinoma of the lung is shown in Fig. 1.29. Those who have smoked for one to nineteen years are down to a non-smoker's risk after ten years of abstention, although the risk seems to be more substantial after longer periods of smoking.

Changing

The results of changes in cigarette type are not as convincing as those of abstention. Mortality ratios are known to be related to cigarette type in the low, middle and high tar ranges (Fig. 1.30). Risks of carcinoma of the bronchus are a little lower in filter cigarette smokers than in non-filter cigarette smokers

(Fig. 1.31) and changing to filters seems to give some protection, although much less than abstention. However, for ischaemic heart disease data from the Framingham study suggests that filters do not offer protection.

Over the last fifty years there have been great changes in the constituents of cigarettes being sold in the United Kingdom (Fig. 1.32) and these changes have accelerated over the last fifteen years.

Part of the reason why changes in cigarettes may not be as beneficial as might be predicted relates to the way they are smoked. The elements of the cigarette which enter the lungs and remain there are dependent upon the volume and frequency of puffs from the cigarette, the depth of inhalation and the

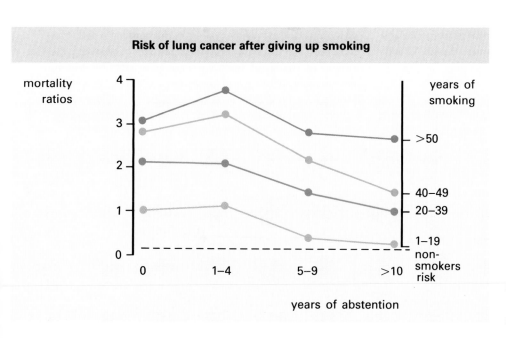

Fig. 1.29 Relative risk of lung cancer in men after giving up smoking according to length of smoking history.

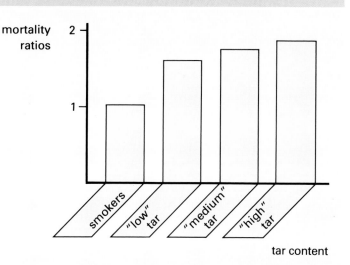

Fig. 1.30 Standardized mortality ratios for cigarette smokers according to the tar content of their usual cigarettes.

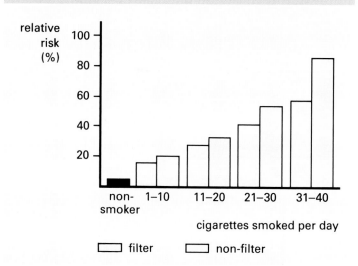

Fig. 1.31 Relative risk of developing carcinoma of the bronchus in smokers of filter and non-filter cigarettes.

timing of these manoeuvres. Smokers themselves are not always very accurate in estimating their inhalation depths but several studies have shown that changes in cigarette constituents result in compensatory changes in the method of smoking. This is shown in Fig. 1.33 in which smokers achieved similar nicotine levels from three very different cigarettes by adjusting their patterns of smoking.

Another way to adjust the product of smoking is to switch to pipes and cigars. Figure 1.34 shows that the mortality figures for pipe and cigar smokers are increased over non-smokers but do not reach the levels of cigarette smokers. Unfortunately they are higher for smokers who switch from cigarettes to cigars and pipes (secondary smokers) than for those who have never smoked cigarettes regularly in the first instance (primary pipe or cigar smokers). This, also, probably relates to the pattern of smoking. Ex-cigarette smokers are more likely to inhale smoke from the pipe or cigar, whereas primary pipe and cigar smokers often do little more than take the smoke into their mouths.

Personal help
Giving up cigarette smoking is difficult and every effort must be made, therefore, to prevent children from starting to smoke.

Nevertheless, there are many patients who want and need to stop smoking. Unfortunately even with anti-smoking advice supplemented with anti-smoking leaflets and follow-up, less than twenty percent of smokers succeed in stopping (Fig. 1.35). However, if all 20,000 GPs in Britain took this approach more than half a million smokers would be expected to stop in one year. Increasing counselling at times of greatest receptivity is likely to increase the chances of stopping, e.g. during pregnancy, at the onset of angina or after a myocardial infarction, if there is a suspicion of lung cancer or on presentation with respiratory symptoms. Nicotine chewing gum (Nicorette) appears to offer more help in the setting of a smoking withdrawal clinic than in general practice, but should be tried in a general approach. Hypnosis and acupuncture have helped some individuals, as have the use of aversion therapy and several other behavioural approaches.

An important part of the process of determining whether an individual has truly stopped smoking, and of assessing the validity of studies of smoking cessation is establishment of non-smoking. In some studies, around one-third of those who claim to be non-smokers have suspiciously high levels of nicotine or carboxyhaemoglobin. Figure 1.36 summarizes the various means available for assessing 'non-smoking'.

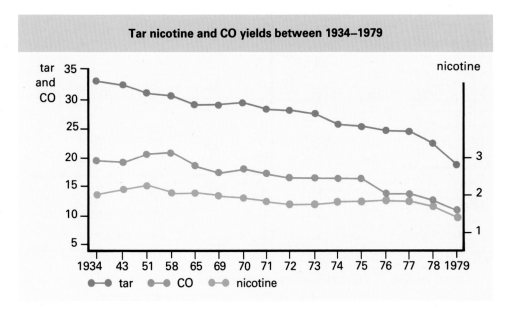

Fig. 1.32 Average tar, nicotine and carbon monoxide yields of UK cigarettes between 1934 and 1979.

Adjustment of smoke exposure to different nicotine content

blood nicotine (mmol/l)

high nicotine | usual brand | low nicotine

Fig. 1.33 Adjustment of smoke exposure by smokers using higher and lower nicotine yielding cigarettes. The grey shaded areas depict the expected nicotine values which would have been achieved if the cigarette had been smoked in the same way as the smoker's usual cigarette. The solid lines are mean achieved levels.

Mortality in pipe and cigar smokers

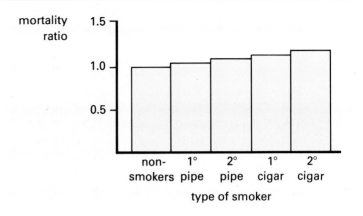

Fig. 1.34 Standardized mortality ratios for pipe and cigar smokers.

Effect of advice on stopping smoking

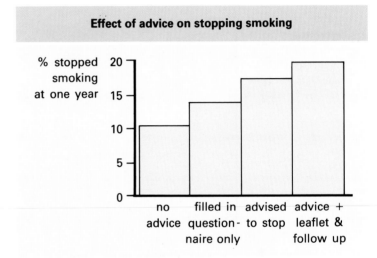

Fig. 1.35 Effect of increasing amount of advice and supplementary help on stopping smoking (figure given for those who had still stopped 1 year later).

Checking validity of 'non-smoking'

Urinary nicotine	clearance dependent on pH; absent after 12 hours tobacco abstention
Carboxyhaemoglobin Expired air carbon monoxide }	half-life one to six hours depending on activity
Serum cotinine Serum nicotine	half-life 30 hours half-life 30 minutes
Serum thiocyanate Salivary nicotine Salivary thiocyanate or iodine }	considerable overlap with non-smokers

Fig. 1.36 Methods of checking validity of 'non-smoking'.

Political help

The politics of tobacco is complex and fraught. The tobacco companies do not divulge their budgets but an idea of the amount spent on cigarette advertising and sponsorship can be obtained when considering that, in 1981, more than £50 million were spent by business on sponsorship of sports and art. The tobacco companies were responsible for the majority of this spending. Compare this to the income coming into ASH (Action on Smoking & Health). ASH depends on the Government for ninety-five percent of its income, which in 1982 was £115,000, for every aspect of its campaign.

Increasing tax on cigarettes causes short-lived reductions in cigarette consumption (Fig. 1.37) but large tax increases would be expected to have a more marked effect. However, the cost benefit of such an approach, in purely economic terms, was deemed by the Government of the day in the 1970s to be politically unwise (Fig. 1.38).

The figures continue to be roughly the same; for 1982 the £2 billion of health service savings resulting from reducing smoking by forty percent is more than 'outweighed' by a loss of more than £4 billion in tax revenue and job losses on the other side of the scales. It has been established that a forty percent fall in cigarette smoking would effectively wipe out all UK tobacco industry profits, although this might be offset to some extent by the industry increasing prices.

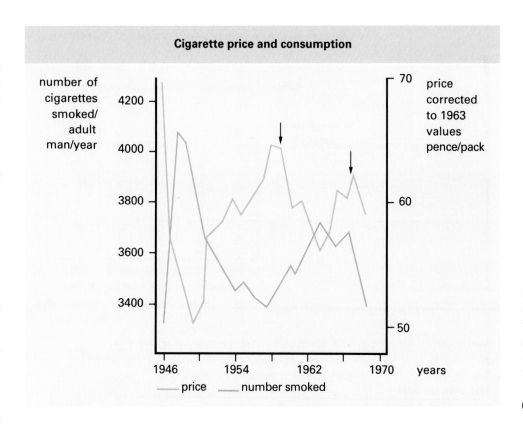

Cigarette price and consumption

Fig. 1.37 Price of cigarettes (corrected to 1963 values) compared to number of cigarettes smoked per adult male per annum. The two arrows indicate the publication of the two reports from the Royal College of Physicians on smoking. (Combined sources)

Economic 'cost' of reduction in smoking

Reduction in smoking by 20% (250,000 premature deaths prevented)	**Reduction in smoking by 40%** (500,000 premature deaths prevented)
DHSS[1] +£12 million by the year 2000	+£29 million by the year 2000
Revenue[2] −£150 million in 5 years	−£305 million in 5 years
Trade deficit[3] −£50 million in 5 years	−£100 million in 5 years

1. Fall in days lost from sickness, balanced by a significant increase in retirement pensions.
2. In 1971 = £1 billion.
3. Saved money spent on imported goods; factory closures.

Fig. 1.38 Economic 'cost' of widespread smoking cessation. (*Smoke Ring: The Politics of Tobacco*, Taylor P. Pub. Bodley Head, 1984.)

2 *Differential Diagnosis of a Mass on the Chest Radiograph*

I.H. Kerr

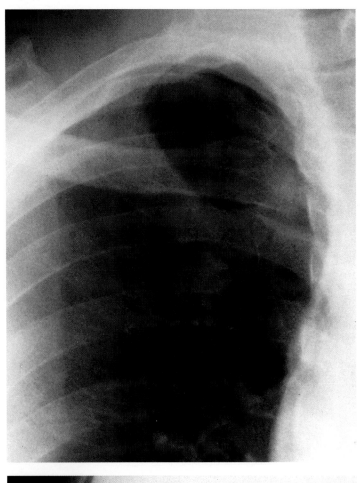

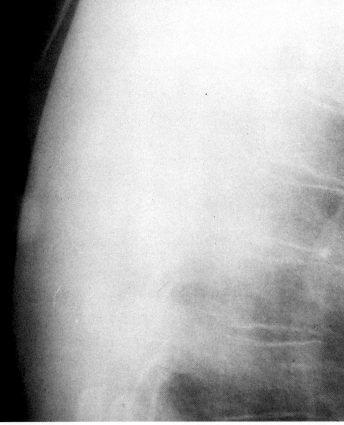

Masses seen on chest radiographs may be diagnosed with some degree of accuracy but it is rare for a lesion to be diagnosed definitively on radiographic appearances alone; examination of bacteriological, cytological or histological specimens usually has to be employed.

There are, however, some helpful general radiological principles which should be employed when a mass is seen on a chest radiograph. The most important investigation when an abnormality is found radiologically is examination of any previous radiographs of the patient; change in appearance of a lesion over a period may provide important evidence as to its nature. Anatomical localization of the lesion should be the first objective, as this will determine the differential diagnoses involved. Is the lesion in the chest wall, pleura, lung or mediastinum? Does the lesion cross anatomical boundaries such as the pleura? If in the lung, is the lesion segmental?

EXTRAPULMONARY MASSES

Tumours of the skin overlying the lungs appear as clearly defined opacities, outlined by air in the same way as are lesions in the lung. If an opacity cannot be seen in the lung in two projections, examination of the skin and chest wall may elucidate the cause (Fig. 2.1). Artefacts, such as buttons on clothing, hair plaits or dressings outside the patients, may sometimes cause opacities over the lung fields. Tumours of the chest wall that cause a mass on a chest radiograph often involve the ribs, and expansion, destruction or displacement of the ribs should be observed (Fig. 2.2). Some extrapleural tumours such as lipomas and neurofibromas (Fig. 2.3) expand inwards, frequently not involving the ribs, and are indistinguishable from pleural tumours. In general, both pleural and extrapleural tumours have smooth medial borders which blend with the adjacent pleura at an obtuse angle.

PLEURAL TUMOURS

Pleural tumours causing localized opacities are rare. Fibromas of the pleura may become very large before discovery. Mesotheliomas spread along the pleura and do not often produce localized pleural masses, though lobulation of greatly thickened

Fig. 2.1 Skin tumour. A well-defined round opacity, apparently in the right upper lobe on the frontal view is seen on lateral view to be due to a small papilloma of the skin on the back.

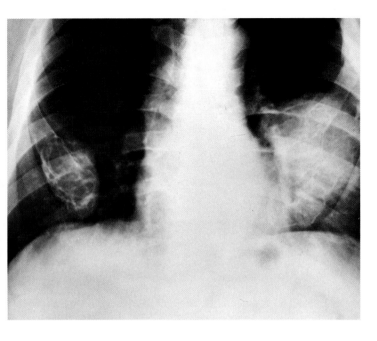

pleura is frequently seen (Fig. 2.4). Loculated interlobar pleural effusions, in either the oblique or horizontal fissures, produce an opacity which may be mistaken for a pulmonary mass. In the frontal view a loculated pleural effusion in the horizontal fissure appears as a round, clearly defined opacity. In the oblique fissure the opacity is clearly defined on its lower margin but is less dense and less well-defined in its upper part (Fig. 2.5, left). Lateral projection shows the lesion to lie in the appropriate fissure. In each case it is oval in shape, with its long axis in the line of the fissure and a 'tail' at each end blending with the fissure (Fig. 2.5, right).

Fig. 2.2 Multiple chondromas of the ribs. The opacity on the right side clearly involves the anterior end of the fifth rib, which is expanded. On the left side, destruction of the anterior ends of the fourth and fifth ribs associated with a mass was due to malignant changes in a chondroma.

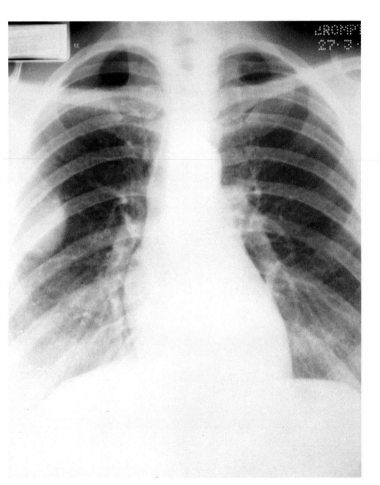

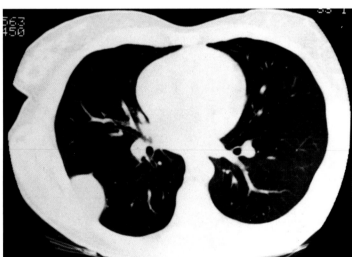

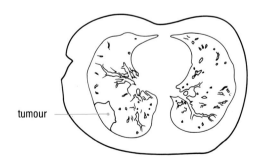

tumour

Fig. 2.3 Neurofibroma of the chest wall. The opacity in the right mid-zone (Left) shows the characteristic well-defined border on one side but a poorly defined outer border of a pleural or extrapleural lesion. The CT scan clearly shows that the lesion is of the pleura or extrapleural tissues.

INTRAPULMONARY MASSES

An intrapulmonary mass on a chest radiograph is an opacity caused by a circumscribed lesion which is not usually confined to normal anatomical boundaries. The causes include congenital and acquired cysts, benign and malignant tumours, and inflammatory lesions, usually chronic. The mass may occlude a bronchus and then be associated with a secondary segmental or lobar infection. Thus, opacities with a segmental distribution are not usually termed masses, but they may be associated with them.

When the air in the alveoli is displaced by an inflammatory exudate, fluid or tumour, a homogeneous or 'ground-glass' opacity occurs. The airspace opacification is of the same density as water and thus obliterates the normal vascular pattern. If the bronchi are patent and still contain air, they can be seen within the opacification; this is termed an air bronchogram. Airspace opacification with an air bronchogram generally indicates an inflammatory condition or alveolar oedema, with the rare exception of a few infiltrating tumours such as bronchiolar cell carcinoma (Fig. 2.6).

Displacement of surrounding structures, such as vessels and fissures, may occur in association with some masses. Displacement away from the lesion is seen in benign lesions, such as cysts; malignant lesions which rapidly infiltrate cause no displacement. Displacement towards the lesion indicates collapse or fibrosis; for example, progressive massive fibrosis (Fig. 2.7).

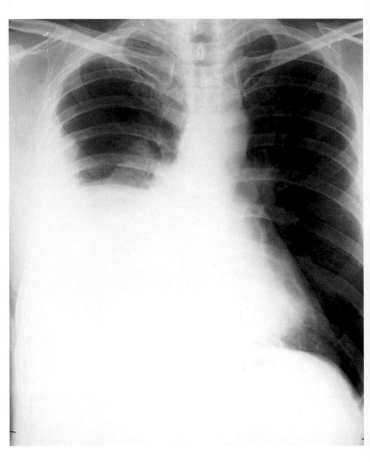

Fig. 2.4 Mesothelioma. There is a lobulated mass attached to the chest wall, with extensive involvement of the lower part of the right hemithorax.

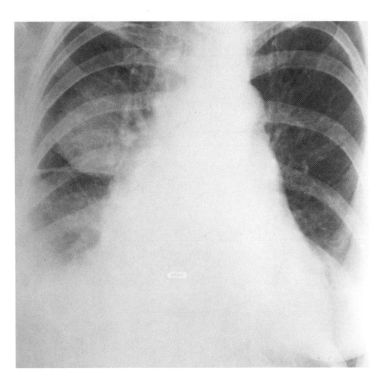

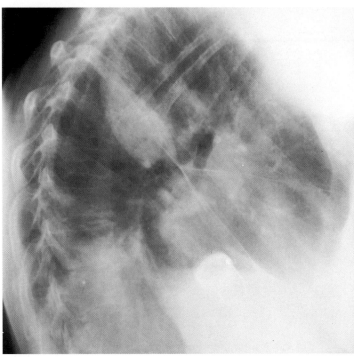

Fig. 2.5 Loculated interlobar effusion. This patient, in heart failure, has a right pleural effusion. The round opacity in the right mid-zone has a sharp lower margin and ill-defined upper margin on frontal view. The lateral view shows the elliptical opacity in the upper end of the oblique fissure.

Calcification

Calcification is seen radiologically in inflammatory masses, and in slow-growing benign tumours. It is a fairly reliable sign of the benign nature of the lesion, though one must remember that both tuberculosis and carcinoma are common diseases and a calcified old tuberculous lesion may be the site of a carcinoma, so-called 'scar cancer'. In the United Kingdom a tuberculoma is the most common calcified granuloma (Fig. 2.8). Other inflammatory granulomas which calcify include those due to histoplasmosis and, rarely, coccidioidomycosis, blastomycosis and ruptured hydatid cysts; the calcification in these cases is laminated or densely punctate, and a small central nidus may

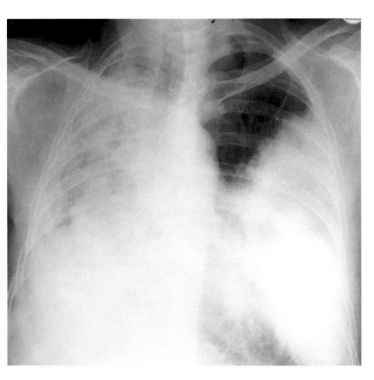

Fig. 2.6 Bronchiolar (alveolar) cell carcinoma. This patient had a lobectomy for carcinoma of the right lung two years previously. Tumour has recurred in the remaining portion of the right lung and also throughout the periphery of the left.

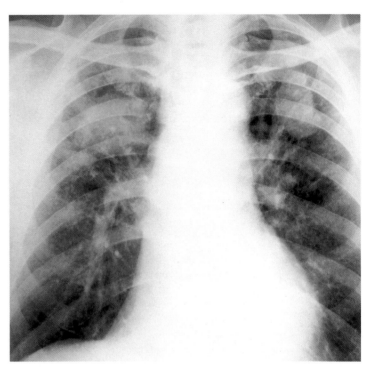

Fig. 2.7 Progressive massive fibrosis. This coalminer, with widespread nodular opacities, developed massive conglomerate shadows in the mid and upper zones due to massive fibrosis. The displacement of the hilar vessels on the right indicates contraction of the lung.

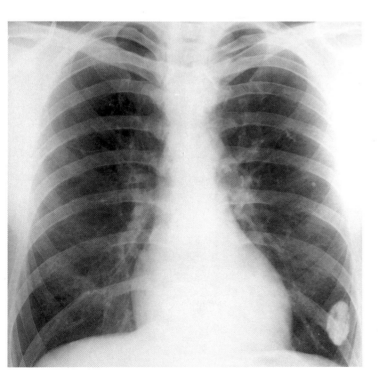

Fig. 2.8 Tuberculoma. Irregular calcification is seen throughout the lesion at the left base. Smaller calcified lesions are also present in the left lung, and there is some calcification of the hilar nodes.

be present. Irregular 'popcorn' or punctate calcification is seen in hamartomas (Fig. 2.9). Amyloid nodules may calcify (Fig. 2.10) but calcification is virtually never seen in rheumatoid nodules (Fig. 2.11) or in Wegener's granulomatosis (Fig. 2.12). Occasionally calcification, or bone, is seen in carcinoid adenoma, and metastases from osteogenic sarcomas may contain calcified osteoid tissue.

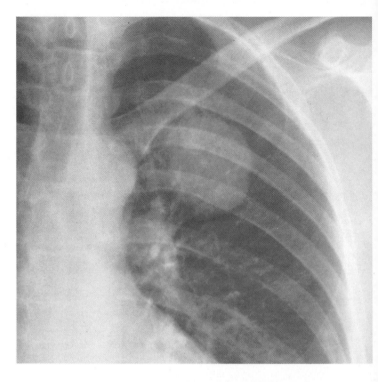

Fig. 2.9 <u>Non-calcified hamartoma.</u> A calcified hamartoma is shown in Fig. 3.70.

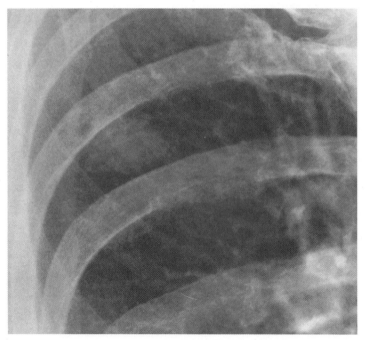

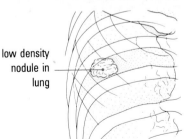

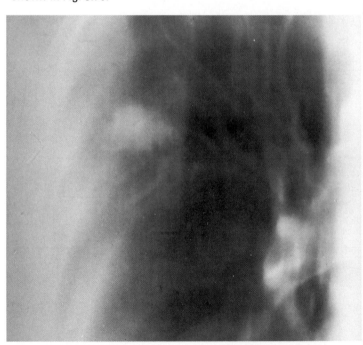

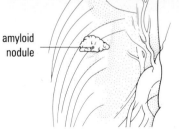

Fig. 2.10 <u>Solitary amyloid nodule.</u> A poorly defined large nodule is visible in the plain radiograph (left). Tomography (right) showed a small central nodule of calcification. The lesion has no specific diagnostic features and its nature was not apparent until biopsy.

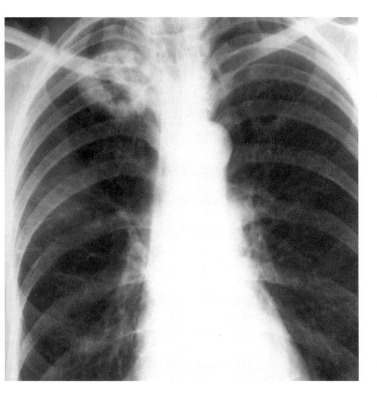

Fig. 2.11 <u>Necrobiotic nodule in rheumatoid disease.</u> In this atypical case, a large cavitating nodule is present in the right upper lobe. Nodules are commonly smaller and may be multiple.

Cavitation

Cavitation is seen in any mass which undergoes central necrosis. It occurs in <u>lung abscesses</u>, <u>tumours</u>, tuberculosis, histoplasmosis, coccidioidomycosis, blastomycosis, rheumatoid nodules, Wegener's granulomatosis, post-traumatic pneumatocele and progressive massive fibrosis, and following pulmonary infarction. Of the tumours which cavitate, squamous cell carcinoma does so most often, though any rapidly growing carcinoma may outgrow its blood supply and undergo central necrosis (Fig. 2.13). The cavity in the neoplasm is often eccentric and irregular, though this is not a reliable differential sign.

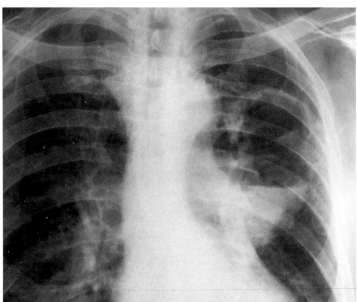

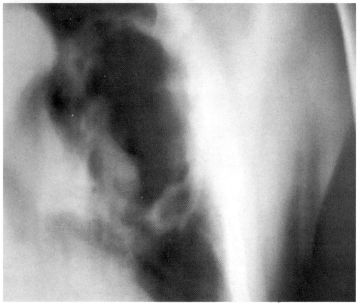

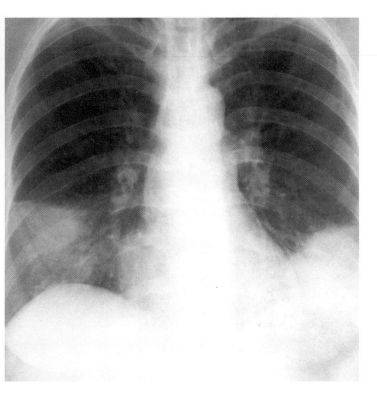

Fig. 2.12 <u>Wegener's granulomatosis.</u> Ill-defined areas of consolidation are seen in the right middle and left lower lobes.

m ost often

Fig. 2.13 Cavitating squamous cell carcinoma. The erect plain radiograph shows a large irregular cavity with a fluid level in the left upper lobe. Tomography (lower) shows an irregular cavity with a mass near the hilum; the fluid level is not seen as the patient is supine.

Cavities may contain fluid when there is liquefaction of necrotic material; this occurs particularly in acute abscesses (Fig. 2.14) but also in some granulomas, such as in tuberculosis. Post-traumatic pneumatoceles often contain fluid. Ruptured cysts may have an air/fluid level; in ruptured hydatid cysts, remnants of the endocyst are seen floating in the fluid — the 'water lily' sign (Fig. 2.15). Necrotic material or blood clot may fill a cavity, and infection by fungus, particularly aspergillosis, produces a central ball of mycelia and fibrin, a mycetoma (Fig. 2.16).

Position

The position of the mass in the lung may suggest a possible diagnosis. Tuberculous infection is commonest in the apex of the upper lobes posteriorly or in the apical segment of the lower lobes, but can occur anywhere in the lungs. Hamartomas (Figs 2.9 and 3.69) are equally common in the upper and lower lobes but are usually within 2cm of the pleural surface. Carcinoid tumours are more frequently central and arise from the larger bronchi (Fig. 2.17). Bronchogenic cysts are also usually central and occur more commonly in the mediastinum (Fig.

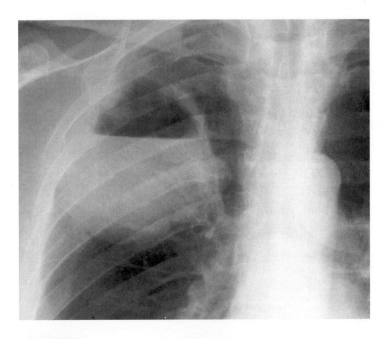

Fig. 2.14 <u>Lung abscess.</u> The radiograph shows a round cavity with a fluid level and a slightly irregular wall. Staphylococci were abundant in the purulent sputum.

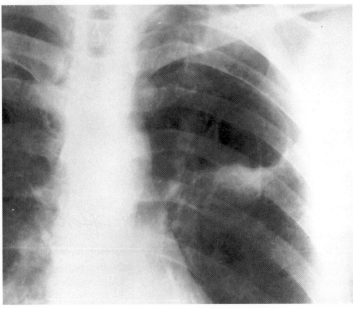

Fig. 2.15 <u>Ruptured hydatid cyst.</u> A thin-walled cavity with a fluid level contains remnants of the ruptured cyst, giving the characteristic 'water-lily' sign.

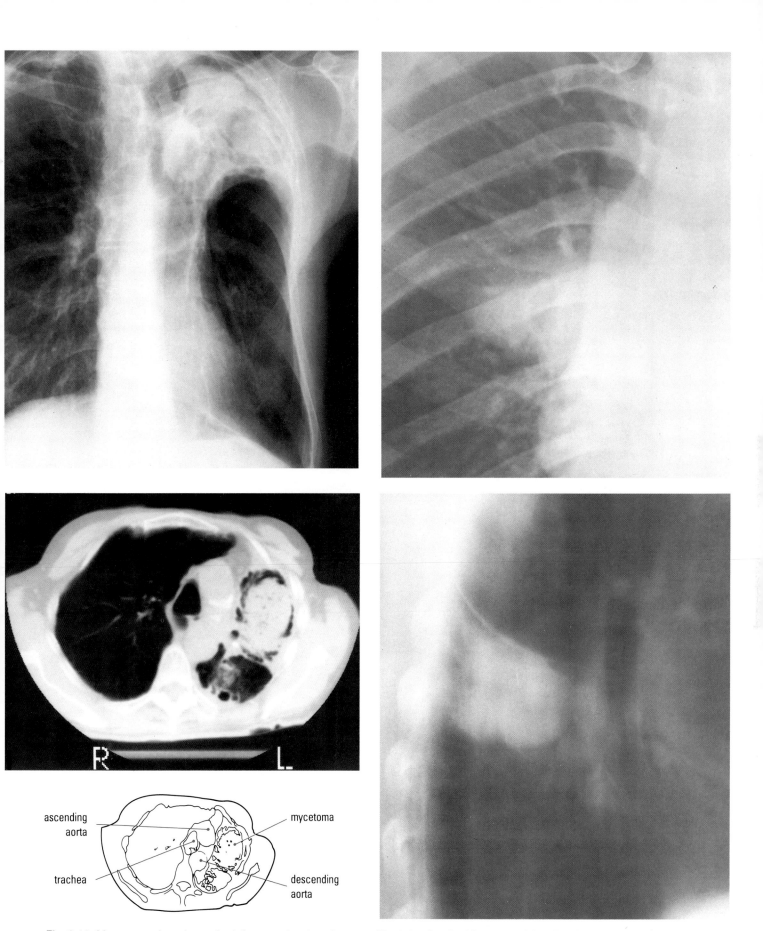

Fig. 2.16 Mycetoma. A cavity at the left apex, the site of previous tuberculosis, contains a 'fungus ball' of *Aspergillus*. The radiograph and CT scan show a crescent of air around the fungus ball.

Fig. 2.17 <u>Carcinoid tumour</u>. A lobulated mass is seen in the apical segment of the right lower lobe, behind the right hilum, in the frontal radiograph (upper) and is clearly defined below the oblique fissure in the lateral tomogram (lower).

ascending aorta

mycetoma

trachea

descending aorta

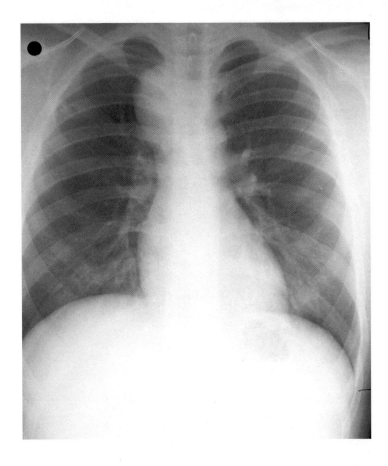

2.18). Intralobar sequestrated segments, deriving their blood supply from the aorta and not the pulmonary artery, are seen posteriorly and medially at the lung base and are twice as common in the left than the right lung (Fig. 2.19). Hydatid cysts are more common in the lower lobes than the upper (Fig. 2.20), as are arteriovenous malformations (Fig. 2.21). Mycetomas, in contrast, are more common in the upper than the lower lobe, since they frequently develop in old tuberculous cavities (Fig. 2.16). Inflammatory lesions are usually confined by the pleura and do not cross fissures or invade the chest wall by direct extension. Actinomycosis (Fig. 2.22) and blastomycosis are the exceptions and may involve the pleura, ribs and intercostal structures or vertebral bodies when there is infection in the lung periphery; the ribs show destruction and

Fig. 2.18 Bronchogenic cyst. This well-defined round smooth opacity on the right of the superior mediastinum is in a typical site, though a retrosternal thyroid would produce the same appearances.

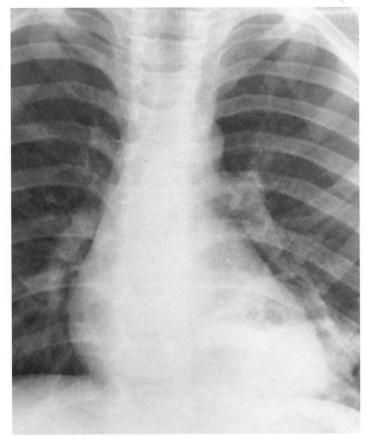

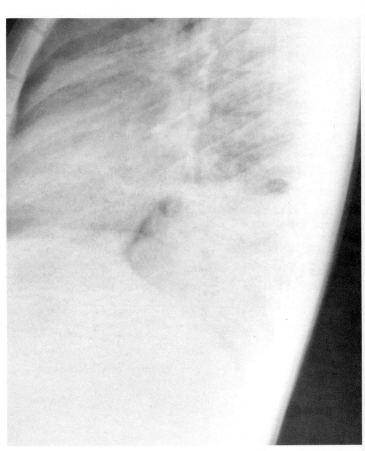

Fig. 2.19 Intralobar sequestrated segment in a child. A cystic lesion with a fluid level is seen in the left lower lobe behind the heart. Some patchy areas of consolidation due to infection are present in the adjacent lung.

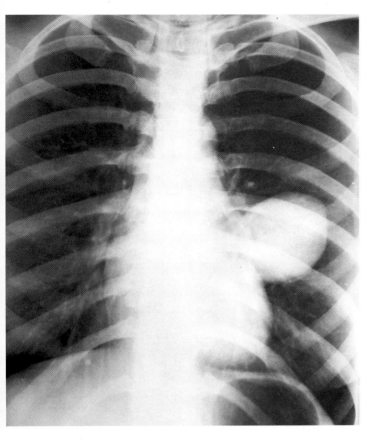

Fig. 2.20 Hydatid cyst. There is a clearly defined smooth round opacity in the upper part of the lingular segment of the left upper lobe. Hydatid cysts are more usually found in the lower lobes.

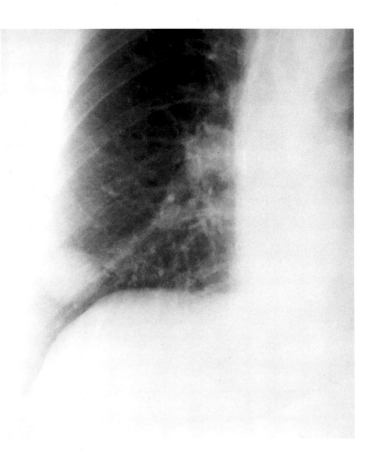

Fig. 2.21 Arteriovenous malformation (fistula). The draining vein and feeding artery cause band shadows between the hilum and heart and the lesion.

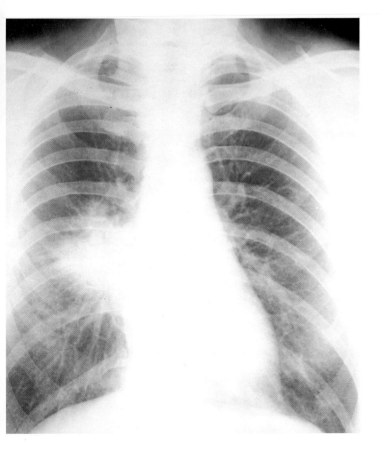

Fig. 2.22 Actinomycosis. An irregular mass at the right hilum, simulating a bronchial carcinoma, is seen to involve all three lobes, crossing the fissures.

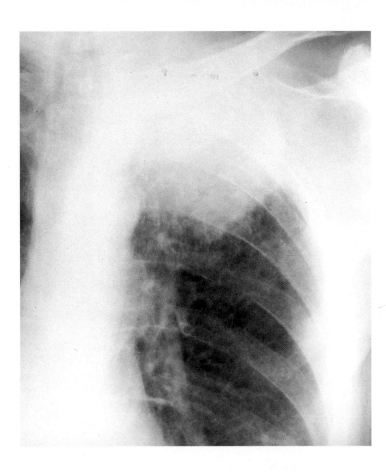

periostitis. Malignant disease frequently crosses the pleural boundaries and involves adjacent lobes of the lung, ribs and vertebrae (Fig. 2.23).

Changes in the normal vessel pattern

These are seen in association with some masses in the lungs. In arteriovenous fistula (Fig. 2.21) a large feeding artery and a large draining vein can be identified running to the hilum.

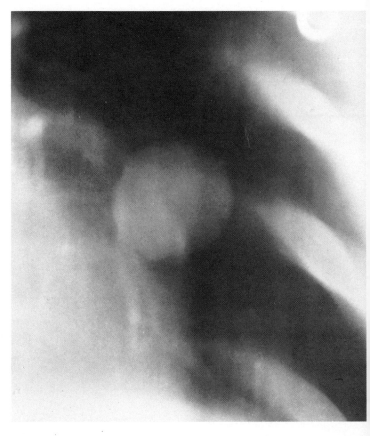

Fig. 2.23 Carcinoma of bronchus. A large mass in the upper part of the left upper lobe has destroyed the posterior parts of the upper five ribs. The tumour has also infiltrated the brachial plexus, giving pain and weakness in the left arm (Pancoast's tumour).

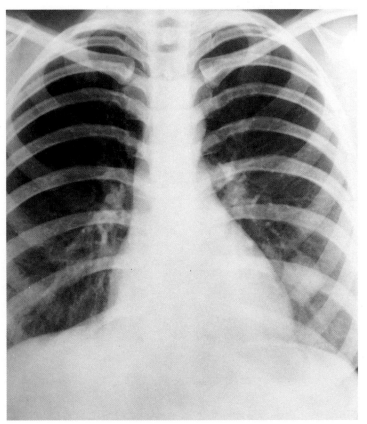

Fig. 2.24 Lymphangioma. This rare benign tumour in the lung has a clearly defined margin and is smooth and round.

Tomography may be necessary to visualize these vessels well and their position can be confirmed by pulmonary arteriography. In malignant disease the pulmonary artery may be invaded by tumour and occluded so that an area of relative avascularity is seen; such an area may also be seen when the bronchus is narrowed, partially blocked by the lesion, due to the reflex constriction of the pulmonary vessels resulting from hypoxia of the affected lung.

Rate of development

Knowledge of the rate of development or growth of a lesion is of considerable value in the differential diagnosis. Lesions which develop over several days are almost certainly inflammatory; lesions which grow only very slowly over several years are more likely to be benign than malignant.

Shape

The shape and margin of a mass are often not as helpful in diagnosis as one might hope. In general, lesions which are clearly defined, smooth, and round or oval are benign (Fig. 2.24), whereas malignant lesions tend to be lobulated with an irregular or spiculate edge. Umbilication of the margin of a round mass has been described as a sign of malignancy, but no one sign is absolutely reliable.

Clinical context

The presence of changes elsewhere in the body, such as hypertrophic pulmonary osteoarthropathy (Fig. 2.25), may be of help in the diagnosis of pulmonary masses. This is most commonly seen in carcinoma of the bronchus, usually squamous cell, and occasionally in adenocarcinoma, but not in oat cell carcinoma. It is also seen in benign fibroma of the lung or pleura. A history of treatment for a primary malignant neoplasm elsewhere in the body suggests that the thoracic mass may be a metastatic tumour (Fig. 2.26), but the possibility of a second primary tumour should not be forgotten, especially if the patient is a smoker. The pulmonary lesion should be fully investigated until its nature is proved.

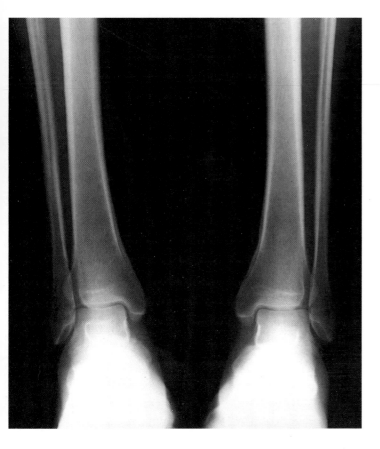

Fig. 2.25 Hypertrophic pulmonary osteoarthropathy. There is periosteal new bone on the medial aspects of both tibias.

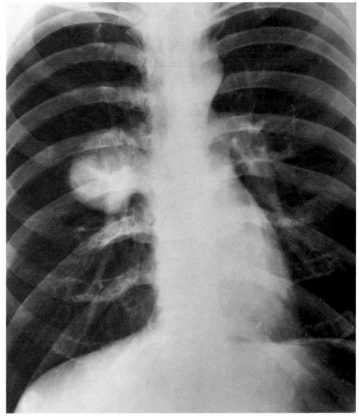

Fig. 2.26 Metastasis. This solitary lesion had no features specific to a metastasis and could have been a primary carcinoma; histology showed it to be a secondary from a previously resected carcinoma of the bowel.

MASSES AT THE HILUM

Masses at the hilum that have irregular margins are usually carcinomas (Fig. 2.27), though occasionally inflammatory masses occur in the perihilar region to mimic central carcinomas. Actinomycosis is one such inflammatory mass (Fig. 2.22) but is rare. Hilar nodes, when enlarged by inflammatory or neoplastic disease, are usually well defined. Bilateral and symmetrical hilar node enlargement is most commonly seen in sarcoidosis (Fig. 2.28). Hilar node enlargement is also seen in lymphoma (Fig. 2.29) but asymmetrical involvement is more common here. Asymmetrical hilar nodes are also seen in tuberculosis, usually in children (Fig. 2.30).

MEDIASTINAL MASSES

Some of the largest masses in the chest arise from mediastinal organs. It may be difficult, on plain radiographs or conventional tomography, to distinguish a mediastinal mass from a mass in the lung adjacent to the mediastinum. Computed tomography (CT) is of immense help in mediastinal lesions. A much more accurate assessment of the origin of various tumours can be made and, with contrast enhancement, vascular lesions such as aneurysms can readily be diagnosed without recourse to arteriography. Arteriography, however, still provides useful information regarding the extent of lesions of the aorta and great vessels, and should be used in hospitals in which CT is not yet available.

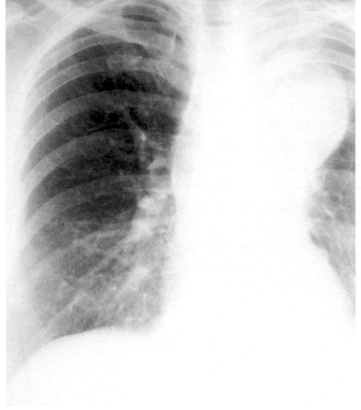

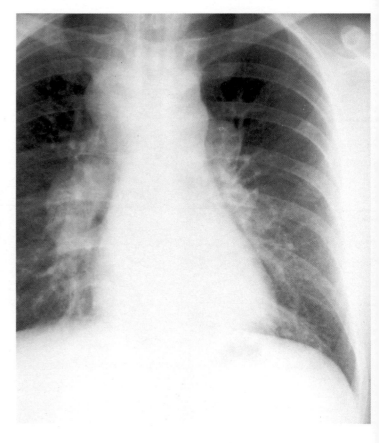

Fig. 2.27 Carcinoma of the left hilum with collapse of the left upper lobe. Note the metastasis in the right sixth rib in the axilla.

Fig. 2.28 Sarcoidosis. There is bilateral hilar node enlargement. A large paratracheal node is seen on the right side of the superior mediastinum. A few small pulmonary nodules can be identified.

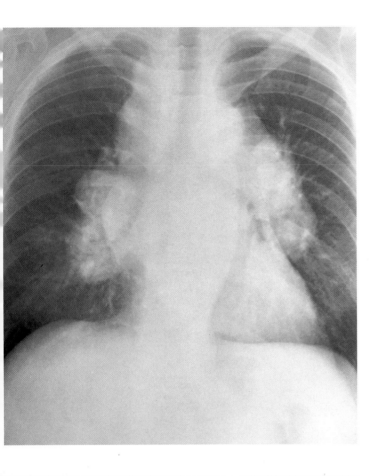

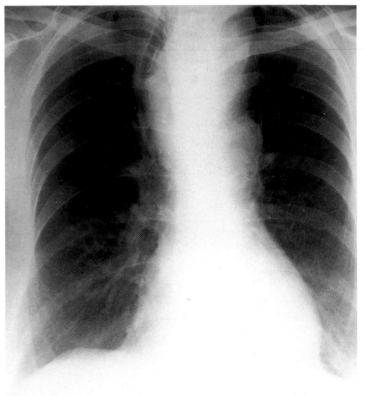

Fig. 2.29 Hodgkin's disease. Hilar and mediastinal lymphadenopathy is present. The nodes in this case are unusually symmetrical and difficult to distinguish from the nodes of sarcoidosis; more commonly the nodes are asymmetrical.

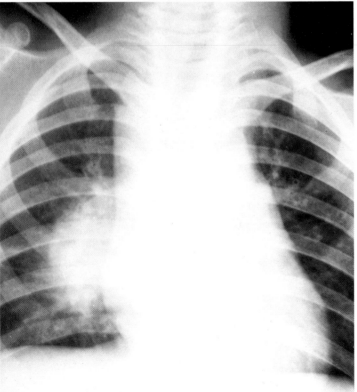

Fig. 2.30 Primary tuberculosis. Enlarged nodes at the right hilum in this three-year-old child are producing a mass. Some patchy shadowing is also seen in the right lower zone and the superior mediastinum is wider than normal.

Fig. 2.31 Retrosternal thyroid. The trachea is deviated to the right and forwards, and also compressed by this retrosternal goitre.

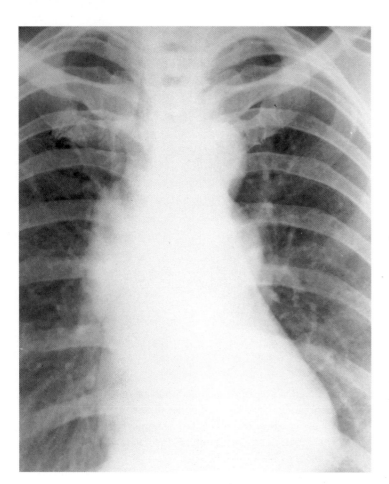

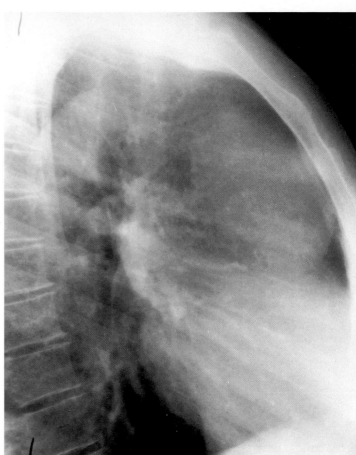

Fig. 2.32 Thymic tumour. A clearly defined oval mass bulging to both sides of the mediastinum is seen to lie behind the sternum on the lateral radiograph.

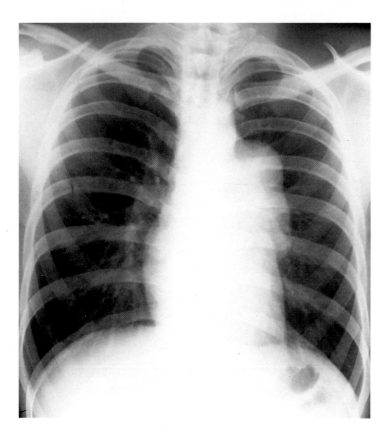

Fig. 2.33 Dermoid cyst. A lobulated, smooth, clearly defined opacity in the anterior mediastinum is bulging towards the left in front of the left hilum, which is seen through it.

The position in the mediastinum of a mass may give a clue to its nature (see Chapter 3). Cystic lesions have clearly defined rounded smooth margins. A retrosternal thyroid (Fig. 2.31) is usually in the superior mediastinum and displaces the trachea to the right or to the left, and either forwards or backwards. The trachea is often compressed by a retrosternal thyroid and this may be so severe as to embarrass respiration. Thymic cysts and tumours (Fig. 2.32) are anterior mediastinal tumours occurring from a level of the upper part of the heart to the level of the arch of the aorta. Some tumours of the thymus are associated with myasthenia gravis and others with severe anaemia. Calcification is often seen in thymic tumours. Thymic lesions

frequently bulge to both sides of the mediastinum on a frontal radiograph of the chest, whereas dermoid cysts (Fig. 2.33), which also occur in the anterior mediastinum, frequently bulge only to one side. Dermoid cysts and teratodermoid tumours may contain calcification, sometimes in the form of a recognizable tooth, and may contain sufficient low-density fat or cholesterol to be detected by CT. Dermoid cysts may become infected and then they increase in size, become less sharply defined on the chest radiograph and give rise to a severe mediastinitis. Other tumours causing masses in the mediastinum include germ cell tumours (seminomas) (Fig. 2.34) and lipomas

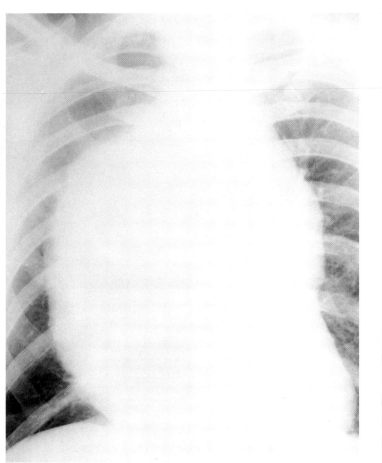
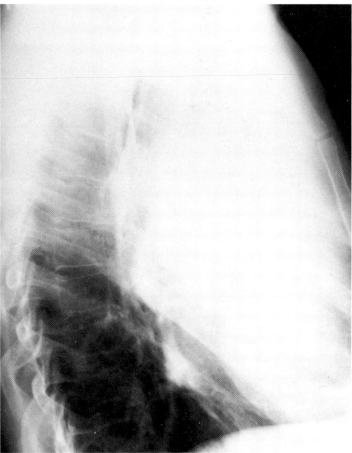

Fig. 2.34 Seminoma. This large retrosternal mass, due to a primary germ cell tumour in the mediastinum, responded dramatically to radiotherapy.

(Fig. 2.35). Pleuropericardial cysts (Fig. 2.36) arise from the pericardium and are seen as clearly defined rounded opacities on the chest radiograph, attached to the heart border on either the left or right side. They do not usually become infected and, though they may increase slowly in size, are extremely benign. They may communicate with the pericardial sac.

Aneurysms of the aorta may be saccular or fusiform (Figs 2.37 and 2.38). They are seen to be continuous with the aortic shadow at some point, though with saccular aneurysms it may occasionally be difficult to identify this connection. The

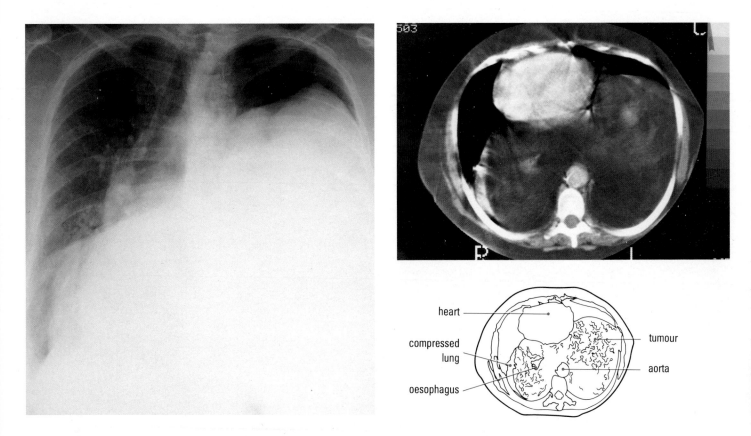

Fig. 2.35 Lipofibrosarcoma. A very large mass obscures the cardiac outline and bulges to both sides of the mediastinum. A left pneumothorax is present following a needle biopsy. The low density of the mass, due to fat, is demonstrated by CT.

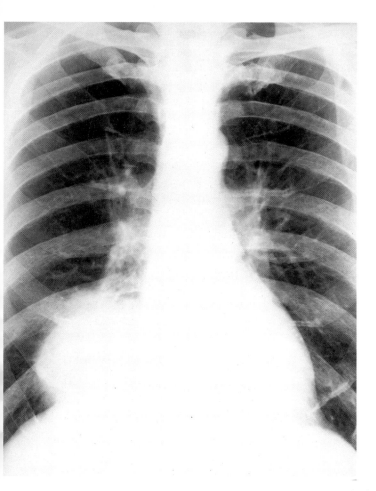

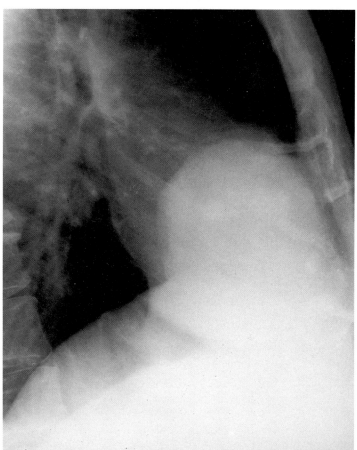

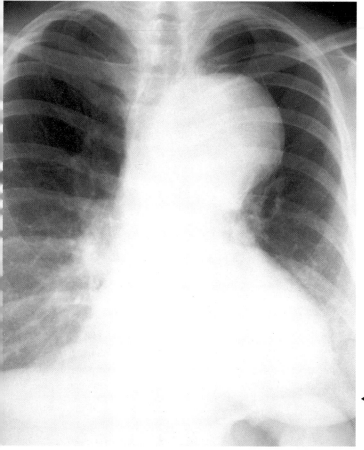

▲ **Fig. 2.36** Pleuropericardial cyst. This cyst lies in the right cardiophrenic angle. The slightly hazy outline is probably due to some compression and collapse of adjacent lung. Differential diagnosis includes a Morgagni hernia (see Fig. 2.40).

◀ **Fig. 2.37** Aneurysm of the arch of the aorta. The aneurysm is causing some compression and displacement of the trachea and left main bronchus. The mass is obscuring the normal aortic arch 'knuckle'.

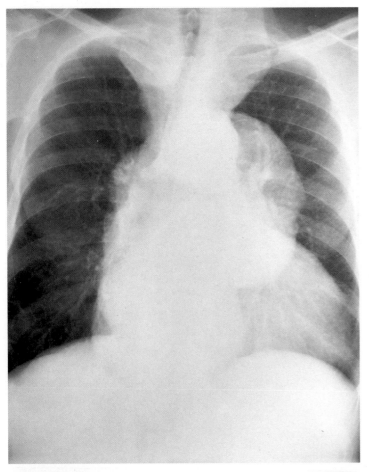

aneurysm is often filled with layers of thrombus (Fig. 2.39) and fluoroscopy to observe pulsation is therefore useless. Most lesions in the mediastinum will transmit pulsation from the great vessels and it is not possible to distinguish transmitted pulsation from expansile pulsation on fluoroscopy. Aneurysms should be diagnosed by CT, radioisotope studies or arteriography and it may be important to do these before other procedures, such as biopsy or thoracotomy, are performed. The possibility that a mediastinal mass is an aneurysm should always be borne in mind. Sometimes an aneurysm will expand into the lung, and bleeding from it can be a cause of haemoptysis. The edge of the aneurysm may in these circumstances become indistinct and the appearances can be confused with a carcinoma of the lung.

Hernia of the diaphragm

Hernia of the diaphragm may give rise to a large mass-like lesion in the chest. Bowel may be present in the hernia, but frequently most of the hernia contains omentum, which has a high fat content, and liver. Hernias of the foramen of Morgagni occur anteriorly, usually in the right cardiophrenic angle, and produce a round swelling arising from the anterior part of the diaphragm (Fig. 2.40). Hernias of the foramen of Bochdalek

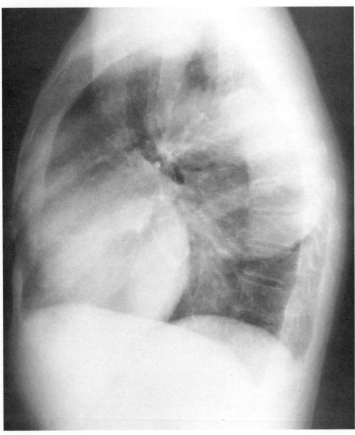

Fig. 2.38 Aneurysm of the descending aorta. In this case the aortic 'knuckle' is visible in front of the mass, but the mass cannot be separated from the shadow of the descending aorta from which it arises.

occur posteriorly and contain kidney, bowel, liver or spleen (Fig. 2.41); they are nearly always seen on the left side. Hiatus hernias are the commonest and produce a mass, nearly always with an air/fluid level, behind the heart, due to the herniated stomach. A barium study will demonstrate a hiatus hernia and late films may show bowel in Bochdalek or Morgagni hernias (Fig. 2.42). Congenital hernias of the diaphragm cause respiratory distress in the neonatal period and may be very large. Rupture of the diaphragm and herniation may occur after trauma.

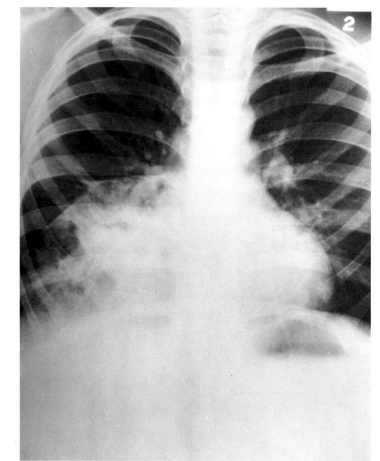

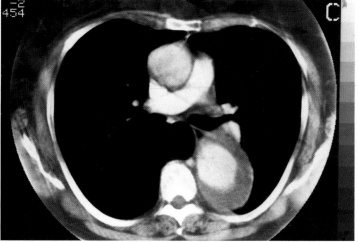

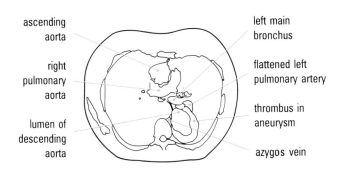

ascending aorta

right pulmonary aorta

lumen of descending aorta

left main bronchus

flattened left pulmonary artery

thrombus in aneurysm

azygos vein

Fig. 2.39 Aneurysm of the descending aorta. This CT scan shows clot within the dilated aorta. Contrast medium enhances the lumen, where there is free blood flow. The left pulmonary artery is adjacent to the anterolateral margin of the aneurysm; the left main bronchus is just in front.

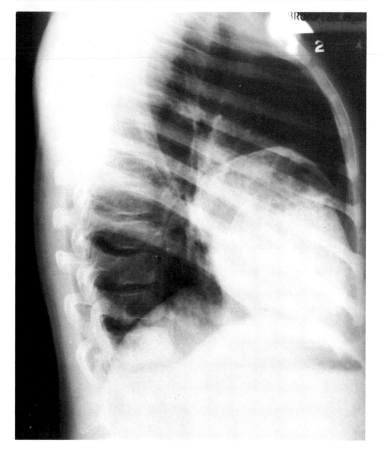

Fig. 2.40 Morgagni hernia. This hernia is filled with bowel which contains gas and faeces. Often only omentum is present.

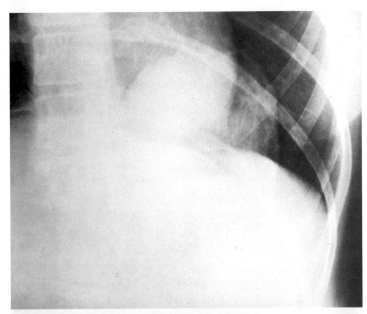

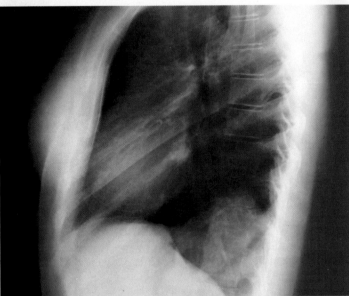

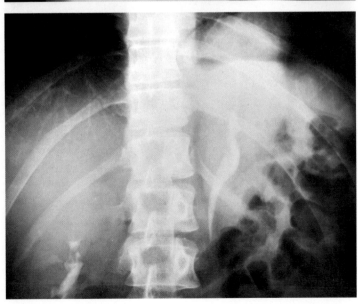

Fig. 2.41 Bochdalek hernia. A bulge is seen arising from the posterior part of the diaphragm behind the heart. The intravenous urogram (bottom) shows that the left kidney lies within this hernia, which also contains perirenal fat.

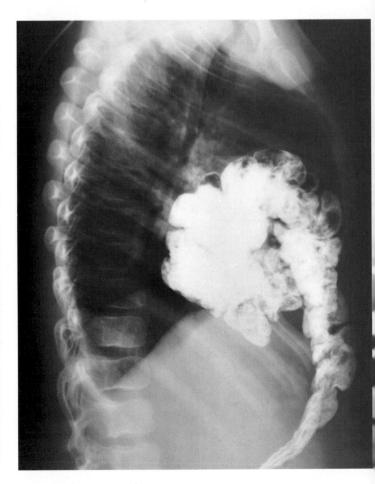

Fig. 2.42 Morgagni hernia. Barium-filled loops of bowel lie in the hernia.

3 *Tumours*

M.E. Hodson and I.H. Kerr

This chapter considers tumours of the trachea, bronchi and distal air spaces; tumours of the pleura and mediastinum are also considered.

Tumours of the trachea are very rare and are usually low grade malignant tumours derived from submucosal glands. They may present with stridor, wheezing, breathlessness or haemoptysis. Secondary malignant deposits in the trachea are also rare.

Malignant tumours of the bronchi are very common but benign tumours also occur. Secondary deposits in the bronchi are rare.

In the distal air spaces primary tumours, such as bronchioloalveolar cell carcinoma, are rare, as are benign tumours. Secondary deposits are common from breast, gut, kidney, thyroid, ovary or testes.

Primary lung tumours	
Malignant (high grade)	Carcinoma of bronchus
	Alveolar cell carcinoma
	Pulmonary lymphoma
	Sarcoma
	Carcinosarcoma
	Pulmonary blastoma
Malignant (low grade)	Bronchial gland tumours
	Carcinoid
Benign	Hamartoma
	Papilloma
	Fibroma
	Leiomyoma
	Lipoma
	Neurofibroma
	Arteriovenous fistula
	Plasma cell granuloma

Fig. 3.1 Primary lung tumours.

Histological types of carcinoma of the bronchus	
Squamous	52%
Oat cell	30%
Adeno	13%
Large cell	5%

Fig. 3.2 Histological types of carcinoma of the bronchus (Huhti 1981).

A classification of primary lung tumours is given in Fig. 3.1. The most common malignancy of the lung, carcinoma of the bronchus, will be considered first followed by a section on other tumours.

CARCINOMA OF THE BRONCHUS

Aetiology

Bronchial carcinoma is the commonest malignancy of males in the Western world. In Britain the mortality rate in adult males is 100 per 100,000. Men are affected more frequently than women but more women are becoming affected as more take up smoking. The predominant age group is fifty to seventy years. The incidence of the main histological types is shown in Fig. 3.2 and a more detailed WHO classification in Fig. 3.3.

All the available evidence points to cigarette smoking as being the major aetiological factor in causing carcinoma of the bronchus. Doll and Hill showed, in 1964, that the incidence among doctors who smoked was much higher than among non-smokers, and the incidence of bronchial carcinoma increased with the number of cigarettes smoked per day (Fig. 3.4). It has also been shown that there is an increased risk in those who smoke pipes and cigars but this risk is not as high as in cigarette smokers (Fig. 3.5). It does however appear that adenocarcinoma and alveolar cell carcinoma are only weakly related to smoking but these histological types form only a small part of the total number of cases.

WHO classification of malignant lung tumours

Squamous cell carcinoma
Variant
1. Spindle cell carcinoma

Adenocarcinoma
1. Acinar adenocarcinoma
2. Papillary adenocarcinoma
3. Bronchiolo-alveolar carcinoma
4. Solid carcinoma with mucus formation

Small cell carcinoma
1. Oat cell carcinoma
2. Intermediate cell type
3. Combined small cell carcinoma

Large cell carcinoma
1. Solid carcinoma without mucin
2. Giant cell carcinoma
3. Clear cell carcinoma

Carcinoids

Mesothelioma

Fig. 3.3 WHO classification of malignant lung tumours.

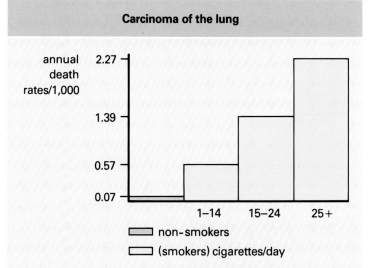

Fig. 3.4 Doll's study of doctors' smoking habits (from Doll and Hill 1964).

Other aetiological factors are of little importance compared with cigarette smoking. It has however been shown that there is a higher mortality in urban than rural dwellers, and a higher incidence of bronchial carcinoma in uranium miners, haematite miners and workers with asbestos (Fig. 3.6), chromates, arsenic and nickel.

Presenting features

Asymptomatic

Up to about five percent of patients with bronchial carcinoma are asymptomatic and are picked up as a result of a routine chest radiograph.

Respiratory symptoms

Haemoptysis is often the first symptom. A patient who has been a heavy smoker and already has some degree of chronic bronchitis will present with slight blood streaking of the sputum.

Cough may have become worse in the patient who already has some degree of bronchitis and sputum volume may have increased.

Chest pain is not so common as haemoptysis or cough but may be pleuritic in nature due to pneumonia extending to involve the pleura; alternatively there may be a deep aching pain due to neoplastic involvement of the mediastinum, or chest wall pain due to involvement of the ribs and intercostal nerves.

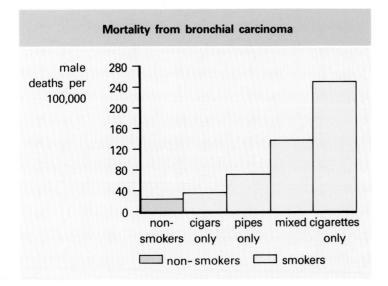

Fig. 3.5 Mortality, bronchial carcinoma, cigarettes/cigars.

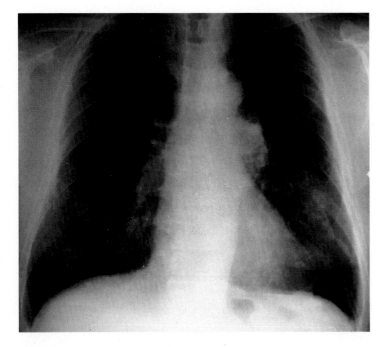

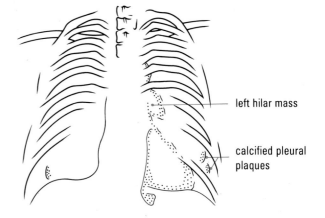

Fig. 3.6 An undifferentiated carcinoma of the bronchus following previous asbestos exposure. A mass is present in the left hilum extending into the apical segment of the lower lobe. Some calcified pleural plaques on both sides are present due to previous asbestos exposure.

Dyspnoea can be present. This may be mild due to a slow increase in the size of the tumour or severe due to pulmonary collapse caused by bronchial occlusion or a large pleural effusion (Figs 3.7 and 3.8). Wheeze and stridor may occur if the tumour involves the large airways. Breathlessness can also be caused by lymphangitis carcinomatosa. The patient may present with pneumonia which fails to resolve after appropriate treatment, the pneumonia having been caused by infection distal to a carcinoma that is obstructing the bronchus. A lung abscess may occasionally form within or beyond the tumour.

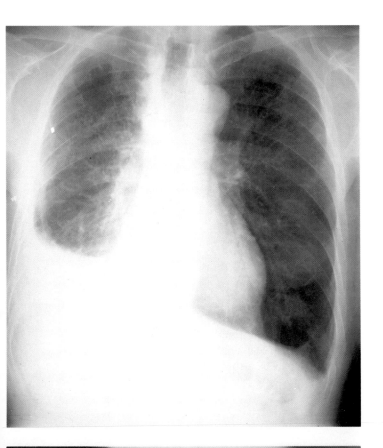

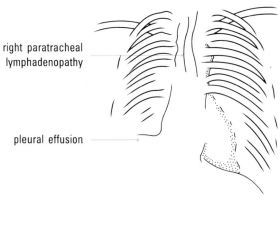

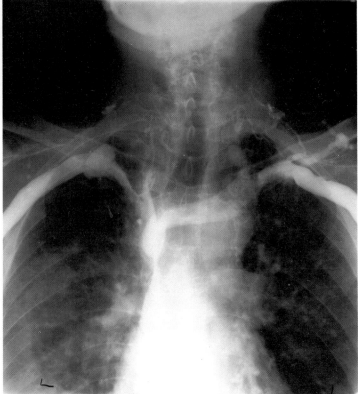

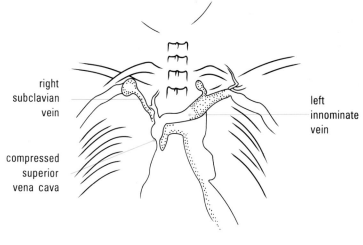

Fig. 3.7 Carcinoma of the right lung showing a right pleural effusion. The right lung is partially collapsed and the right paratracheal lymph nodes are enlarged causing widening of the superior mediastinum. The superior vena cavagram (below) shows compression of the superior vena cava from the right at the level of the carina by lymph node involvement.

47

General symptoms

The patient may present with loss of weight, anorexia, tiredness or unexplained pyrexia.

Symptoms due to metastases

Common symptoms of cerebral metastases include headaches, fits, personality changes and occasionally hemiplegia. Patients presenting with jaundice may have liver metastases and bone

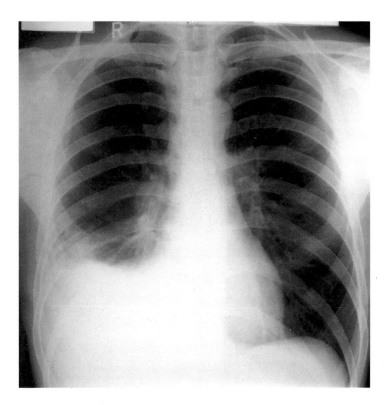

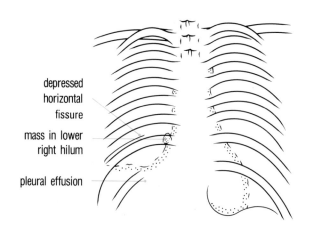

Fig. 3.8 Adenocarcinoma of the bronchus with a right pleural effusion. There is a mass in the lower right hilum with collapse and consolidation of the right middle, and left lower, lobes. The effusion was blood-stained on aspiration.

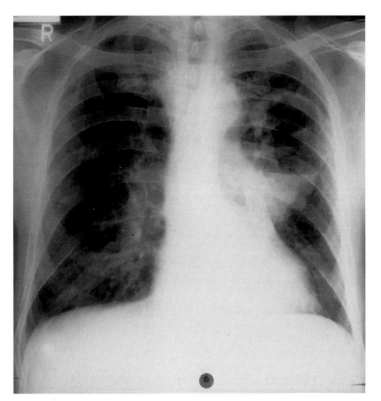

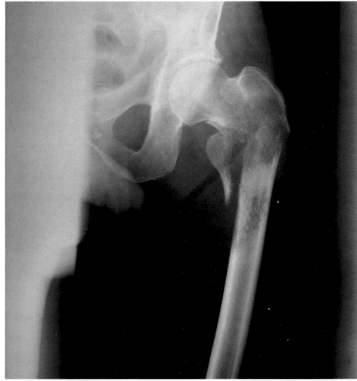

Fig. 3.9 A large cavity in the left lung with a fluid level due to a cavitating carcinoma. Radiograph of the left hip and femur in the same patient show a pathological fracture due to metastases causing destruction of the lesser trochanter.

pain may be due to secondary deposits (Fig. 3.9).

Axillary lymphadenopathy is rare and occurs only if the tumour has invaded the chest wall. The patient may present with an enlarged lymph node in the cervical region.

Symptoms due to extension of the tumour

Chest wall involvement causes pain in the chest wall as ribs and intercostal nerves are invaded by the tumour.

Pleural effusion is caused by tumour involving the pleura, is characteristically blood stained and frequently reaccumulates after aspiration.

Nerve involvement can manifest itself in several ways:

1. Involvement of the phrenic nerve will produce paralysis of the hemidiaphragm on the affected side and this may cause dyspnoea.
2. Invasion of the left recurrent laryngeal nerve causes hoarseness.
3. A Pancoast's tumour (Fig. 3.10) is the name given to a tumour at the apex of the lung. It may involve the cervical sympathetic trunk, causing a Horner's syndrome, or the brachial plexus, giving pain, paraesthesia and weakness in the upper limb. It may also erode the ribs.

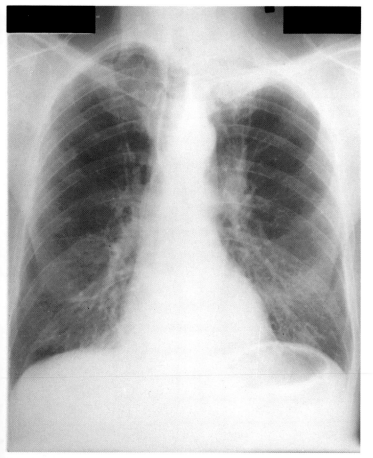

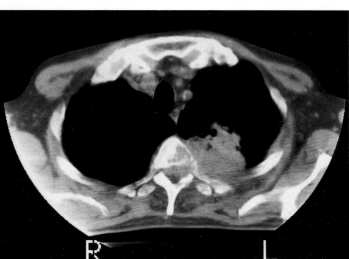

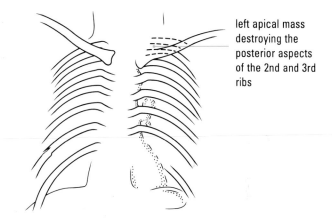

left apical mass destroying the posterior aspects of the 2nd and 3rd ribs

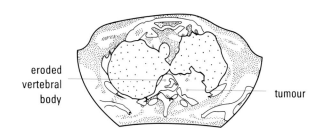

eroded vertebral body

tumour

Fig. 3.10 Pancoast's tumour. There is a mass at the left apex on the frontal view. Close inspection shows destruction of the posterior half of the second rib and part of the third rib. CT section through the tumour shows its proximity to the posterior ends of the ribs and partial destruction of the ribs and adjacent vertebral body.

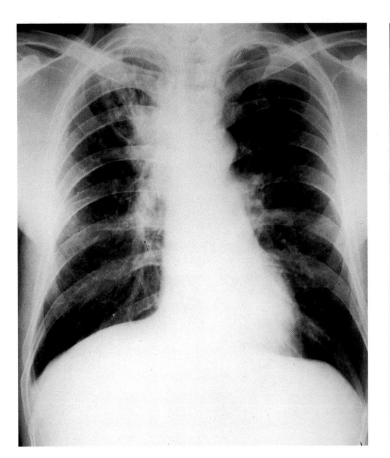

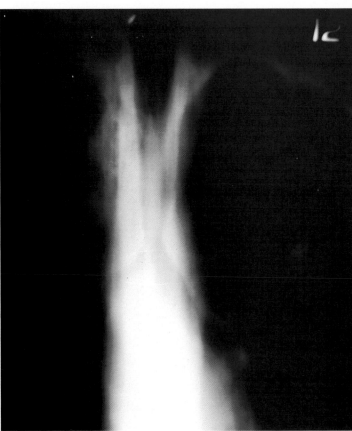

Fig. 3.11 A mass in the right upper lobe adjacent to the mediastinum. Tomograph of the trachea shows narrowing of the lower end of the trachea and right main bronchus.

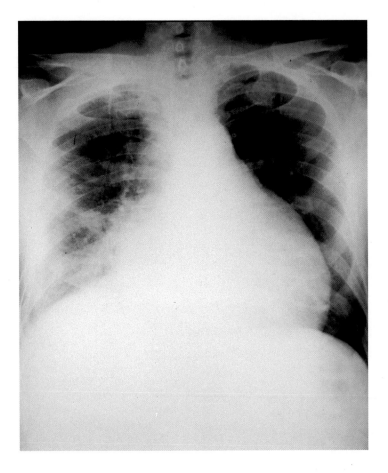

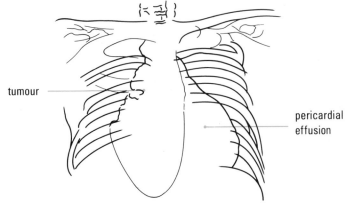

Fig. 3.12 Small cell tumour. Carcinoma of the right lung has involved the pericardium leading to a pericardial effusion.

4. Stridor is uncommon and may be due to obstruction of the trachea or main bronchus by carcinoma (Fig. 3.11).

Dysphagia is due to oesophageal obstruction by the tumour.

Pericardial involvement (Fig. 3.12) can cause a blood-stained pericardial effusion that results in compression of the heart (cardiac tamponade). It may also cause cardiac arrhythmias.

Superior vena cava obstruction is the result of compression of the superior vena cava by tumour invading the mediastinum (Figs 3.13 and 3.14). The patient is usually very distressed, with swelling and cyanosis of the face and neck and there is oedema of the arms. The veins on the neck and upper part of the chest are dilated.

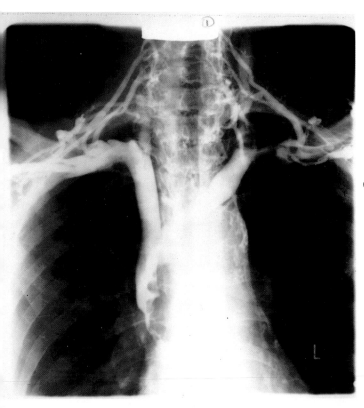

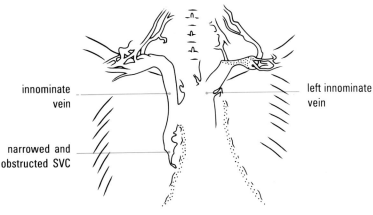

Fig. 3.13 Superior vena cavagram showing obstruction of the superior vena cava due to carcinoma of the bronchus.

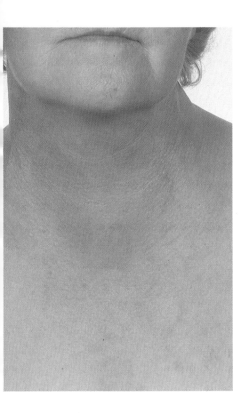

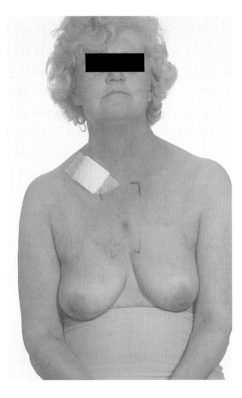

Fig. 3.14 Small cell tumour causing superior vena caval obstruction; the diagnosis was confirmed by biopsy of a supraclavicular lymph node.

Lymphangitis carcinomatosa may be unilateral or bilateral and often causes severe breathlessness (Figs 3.15 & 3.16).

Features due to non-metastatic syndromes

Finger clubbing (Fig. 3.17) and hypertrophic pulmonary osteo-arthropathy (Fig. 3.18) are characterized by pain and swelling of the joints of the fingers, wrists and ankles. A radiograph will show new periosteal bone formation at the distal ends of the bones of the forearm and leg. Neuromuscular syndromes include myopathy, neuropathy, myasthenia gravis-like syndromes, dementia and cerebellar degeneration.

Endocrine syndromes are most commonly associated with small cell tumours. Hypercalcaemia may cause thirst, polyuria, constipation or confusion. A patient may present with Cushing's syndrome due to ectopic ACTH production; inappropriate ADH secretion or ectopic parathormone production leading to hyponatraemia and hypercalcaemia respectively. Abnormalities of sugar metabolism causing hyper- or hypoglycaemia have

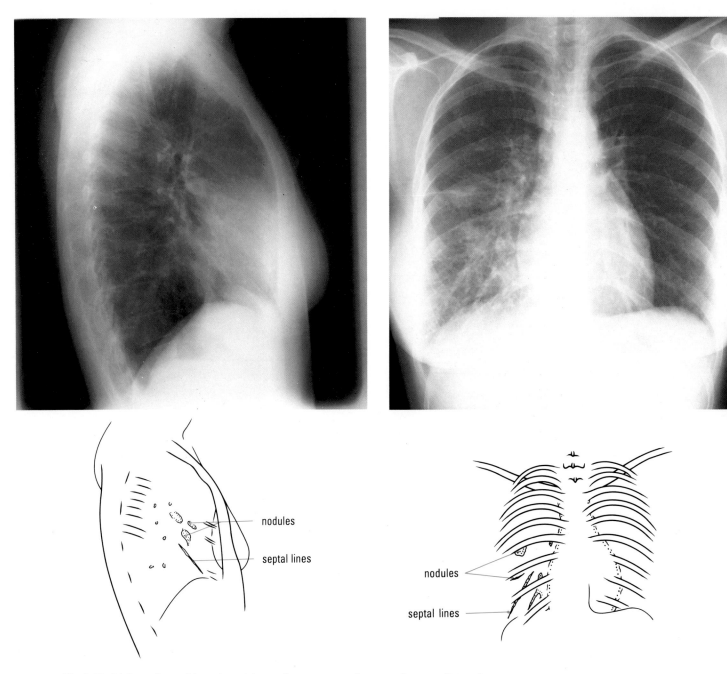

Fig. 3.15 Right unilateral lymphangitis carcinomatosa, primary unknown. Extensive shadowing, predominantly linear, is seen in the right lung. Prominent septal lines are present and a few nodules of varying sizes are also present in the right lower zone. The left lung is clear.

also been reported, as well as hyperthyroidism, red cell aplasia and gynaecomastia. Nephrotic syndrome is a very rare complication and is thought to be due to the deposition of tumour antigens giving rise to immune complex mediated disease.

Migratory thrombophlebitis of the superficial veins occasionally occurs.

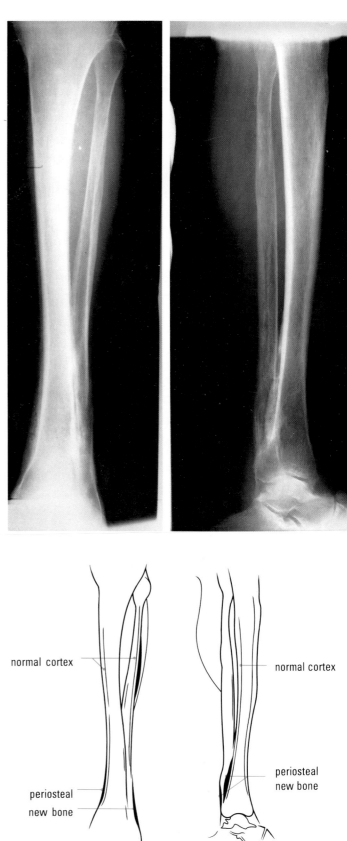

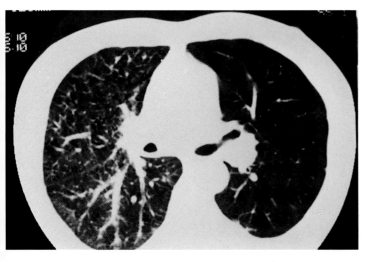

Fig. 3.16 High resolution CT (3mm slice) in right-sided lymphangitic carcinomatosis showing thickening of the septa, and bronchovascular bundles. Compare the appearances of the right lung with that of the left.

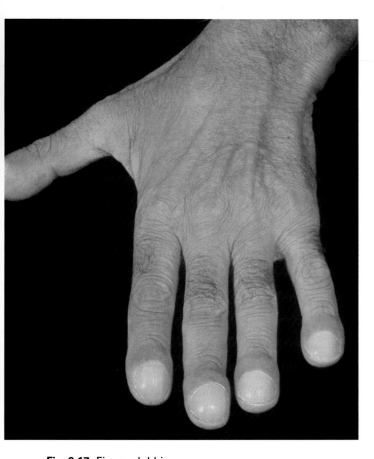

Fig. 3.17 Finger clubbing.

normal cortex

normal cortex

periosteal
new bone

periosteal
new bone

Fig. 3.18 Tibia and fibula of a patient with squamous cell carcinoma of bronchus showing marked periosteal new bone formation secondary to hypertrophic pulmonary osteoarthropathy.

Physical examination

Finger clubbing is present in many patients with a bronchial carcinoma. Other physical signs depend on the severity of the disease. There may be no abnormal signs. There may be the physical signs of pneumonia, collapse, pleural effusion, or of the tumour mass itself. Over the tumour there may be dullness to percussion and reduced air entry. There may be a fixed rhonchus when the tumour is obstructing a major airway.

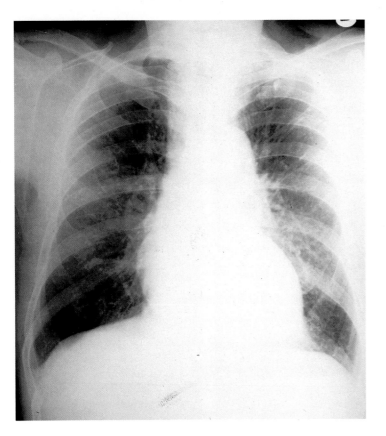

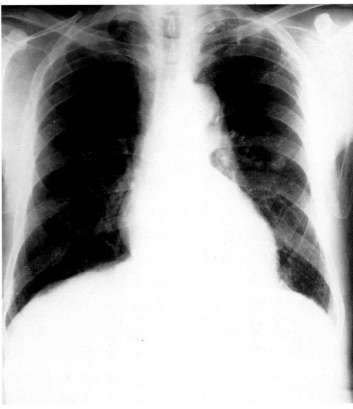

Fig. 3.19 Old calcified lesion (left) at the left apex. The mid-lung field is clear. One year later (right). A nodule without symptoms; this proved to be a carcinoma of the bronchus.

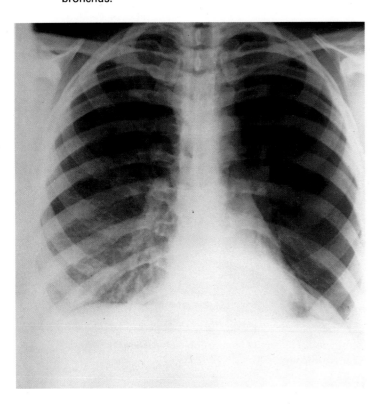

Fig. 3.20 Carcinoma of the bronchus showing obstructive overinflation (obstructive emphysema). The left lung shows decreased vascularity but no definite mass can be identified. There is a carcinoma of the left main bronchus. On expiratory film there was air trapping in the left lung.

Local metastases may cause tenderness of ribs or long bones, cervical lymphadenopathy, jaundice or signs of superior vena cava obstruction.

Investigations

The object of investigations is to discover if the patient has a carcinoma and, if so, its histology and operability.

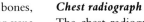

Chest radiograph

The chest radiograph may initially be normal (Fig. 3.19) or show no definite mass (Fig. 3.20) but any of the following may occur:

A solitary nodule or 'coin' lesion of any size may be present (Fig. 3.21). An opacity with an irregular margin adjacent to the hilum is a very common radiological appearance (Fig. 3.22)

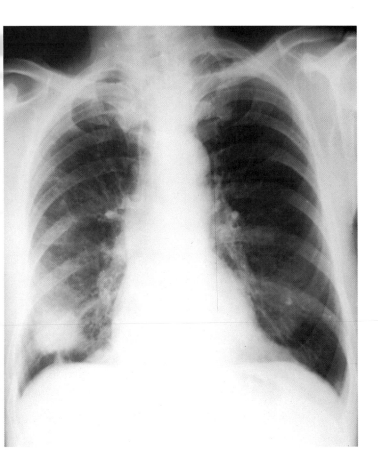

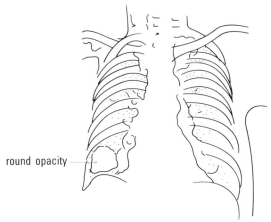

round opacity

Fig. 3.21 Squamous cell carcinoma, peripheral round opacity.

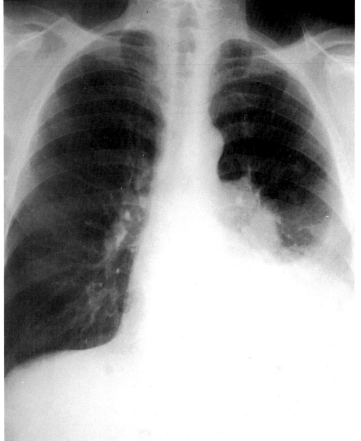

Fig. 3.22 Oat cell carcinoma with effusion: mass at the left hilum with a left pleural effusion.

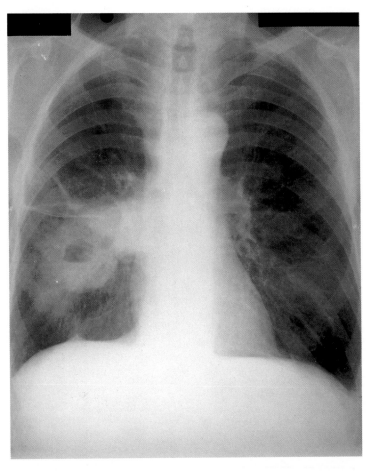

— this can be caused by the tumour itself or by metastases to the hilar lymph nodes. Cavitating lesions may be present (Fig. 3.23). The collapse of a lobe or a whole lung (Figs 3.24–3.26) may be present with the signs of mediastinal displacement. The appearance may be of pneumonia distal to a still relatively small carcinoma. Lymphangitis carcinomatosa causes linear shadows which may be unilateral or bilateral (Fig. 3.27). Pleural effusion can be present. Bony metastases involving the rib cage can occur. The mediastinum may be widened due to lymph node metastases. Elevation of the hemidiaphragm due to a phrenic nerve palsy (Fig. 3.28) is possible and multiple pulmonary metastases can occur.

Fig. 3.23 Cavitating carcinoma of the bronchus in a patient with coal miners' pneumoconiosis. There is lymph node involvement at the right hilum.

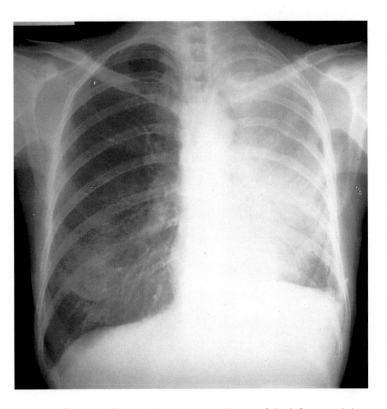
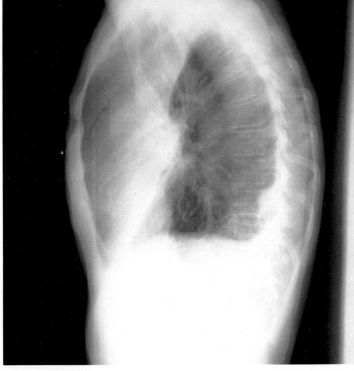

Fig. 3.24 Frontal view shows collapse of the left upper lobe. Posterior part of the left sixth rib shows an area of destruction. The lateral view shows a pleural nodule posteriorly above the diaphragm.

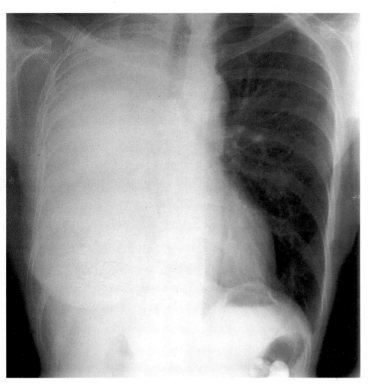

Fig. 3.25 Squamous cell carcinoma of the bronchus: total collapse of the right lung. There is occlusion of the right main bronchus at its origin and narrowing of the left main bronchus. A left mastectomy had previously been performed for carcinoma.

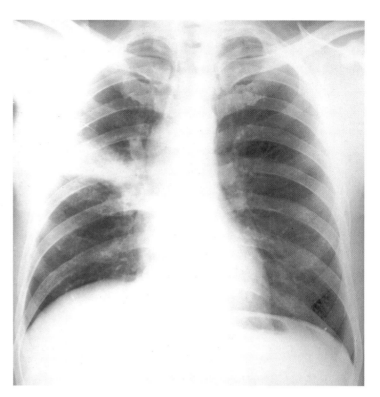

Fig. 3.26 Squamous cell carcinoma of the bronchus: collapse and consolidation in the anterior segment of the right upper lobe with a mass at the right hilum. A large node is present in the right tracheobronchial angle.

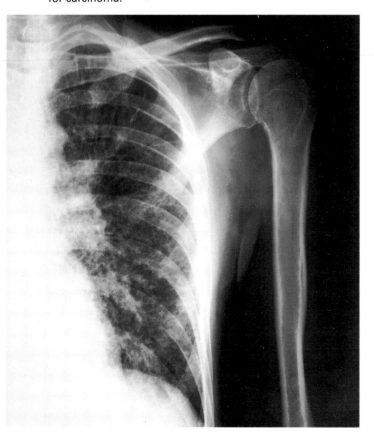

Fig. 3.27 Lymphangitis carcinoma. Reticulonodular shadows in the left lung are due to lymphatic permeation by carcinoma.

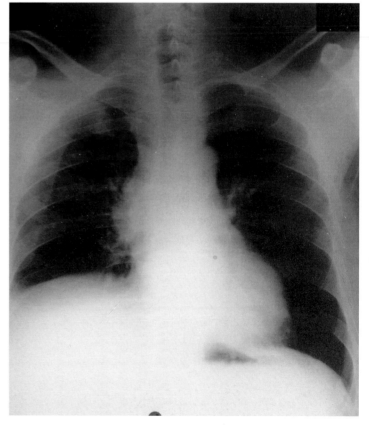

Fig. 3.28 Carcinoma of the bronchus with right phrenic nerve paralysis. A mass is present at the right hilum and there is elevation of the right dome of the diaphragm.

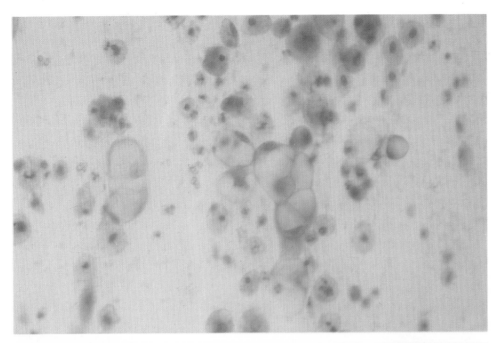

Fig. 3.29 Adenocarcinoma cells in sputum. Vacuolation of the cytoplasm indicates mucus synthesis and hence glandular differentiation.

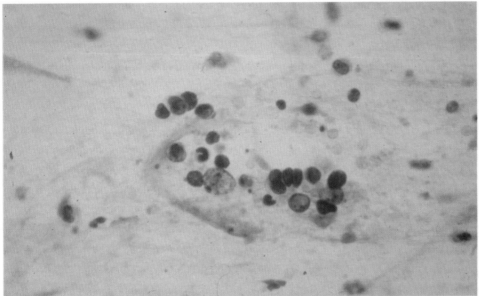

Fig. 3.30 Small cell carcinoma cells in sputum. The dense nuclear chromatin, very sparse cytoplasm and moulding of adjacent nuclei where the cells are in contact are characteristic of this type of tumour.

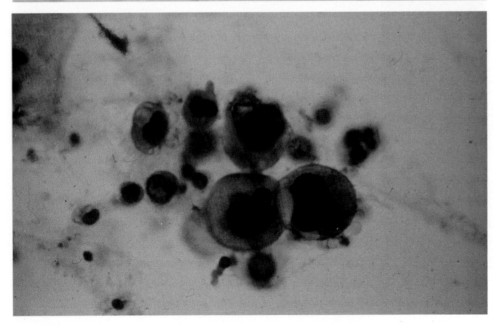

Fig. 3.31 Squamous carcinoma cells in sputum. The cytoplasm of these cells is plentiful and eosinophilic due to keratinization, whilst the nuclei show the atypia and pleomorphism characteristic of malignancy.

Sputum cytology

This is a very useful examination if proper specimens are obtained and an experienced cytologist is available. Three early morning specimens obtained before the patient has eaten should be examined for malignant cells. In over eighty percent of patients with lung cancer this test is positive (Figs 3.29–3.31).

Bronchoscopy

In the majority of patients the diagnosis can be made by bronchoscopy (Fig. 3.32) but peripheral tumours are not visible bronchoscopically. The fibreoptic instrument allows this procedure to be done under a local anaesthetic and a biopsy to be obtained (Figs 3.33–3.37). At the same time attention is

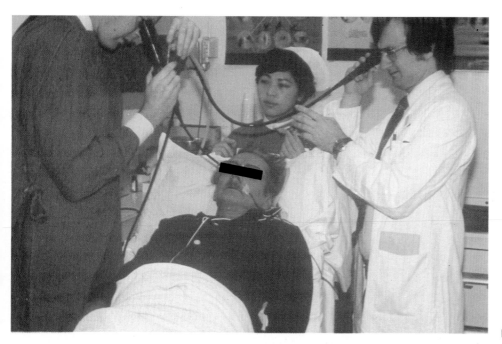

Fig. 3.32 Fibreoptic bronchoscopy.

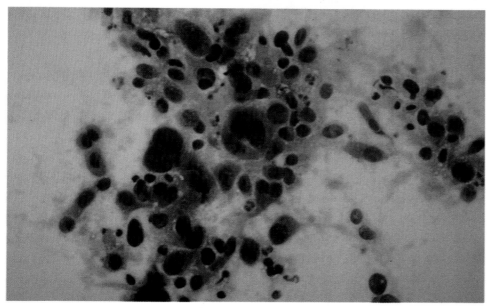

Fig. 3.33 Large cell carcinoma cells in a bronchial brushing. These cells have pleomorphic nuclei that lack the denseness seen in small cell carcinoma, and a moderate amount of cytoplasm that lacks evidence of mucus storge or keratinization.

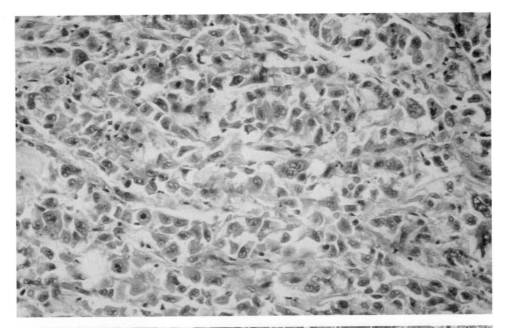

Fig. 3.34 Histology, large cell carcinoma. Cells similar to those seen in Fig. 3.33 are arranged in sheets in this tissue section.

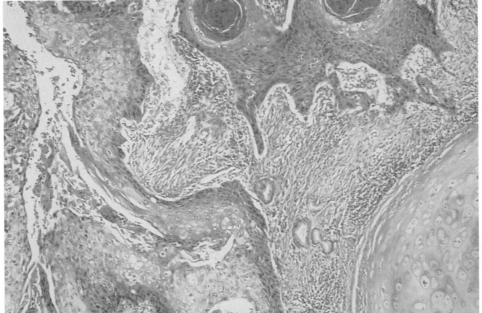

Fig. 3.35 Histology, squamous cell carcinoma. Bands of tumour cells show stratification and keratinization with the formation of distinctive keratin 'pearls'. Bronchial cartilage can be recognized (lower right).

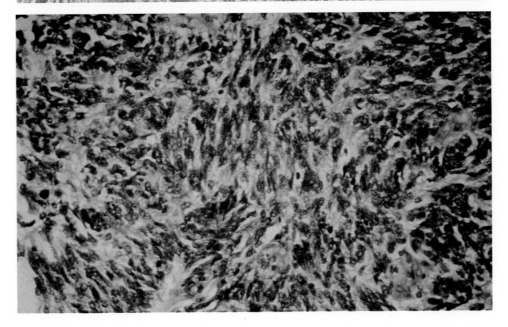

Fig. 3.36 Histology, small cell carcinoma consisting of spindle or 'oat'-shaped cells with dense nuclei and very sparse cytoplasm.

paid to the movement of the vocal cords and the shape of the carina. If the vocal cords are paralysed due to recurrent laryngeal involvement or the main carina widened — indicating metastases to the subcarinal lymph nodes — the tumour is inoperable.

Pleural aspiration

If pleural fluid is present this should be aspirated and examined for malignant cells. At the same time a pleural biopsy should be performed using an Abram's needle. The effusion is usually blood-stained if the pleura is invaded by tumour. Reactive effusions can occur without malignant cells involving the pleura.

Percutaneous needle biopsy

This is carried out under fluoroscopic control. It is particularly useful for peripheral tumours not accessible to the fibreoptic bronchoscope (Fig. 3.38).

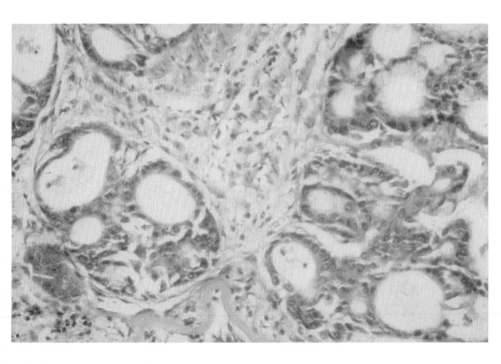

Fig. 3.37 Histology, adenocarcinoma showing prominent glandular differentiation.

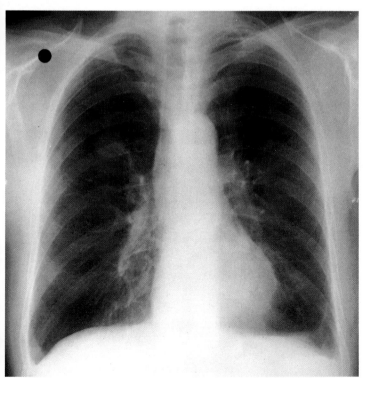

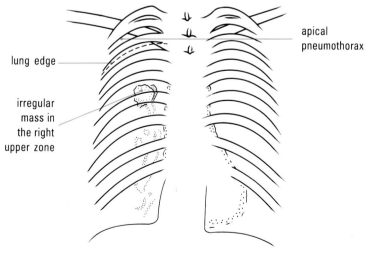

Fig. 3.38 A slightly irregular opacity in the right upper zone with no specific radiological features. A small pneumothorax is present following needle aspiration and biopsy.

Lymph node biopsy

Enlarged cervical or scalene nodes should be biopsied.

Mediastinoscopy

This may be carried out before thoracotomy in a patient with known bronchial carcinoma. If there are metastases in the mediastinal lymph nodes the tumour is inoperable and thoracotomy can be avoided.

Barium swallow

If a patient has dysphagia a barium swallow is indicated to see if there is enlargement of mediastinal nodes pressing on the oesophagus (Fig. 3.39).

Screening of the diaphragm

Involvement of the phrenic nerve by tumour can cause paralysis of the diaphragm which can be confirmed by screening (Fig. 3.40).

Computerized tomography (CT)

CT scan of the thorax will help to determine the extent of the tumour, identifying lymphadenopathy or the presence of metastases in the chest (Figs 3.41–3.45). It should be noted that enlargement of the lymph nodes does not necessarily indicate that they are invaded by tumour.

Diagnostic thoracotomy

In the majority of patients the above investigations will confirm the presence or absence of a carcinoma and its histology. Occasionally however a diagnostic thoracotomy may be necessary.

Other investigations

Once it has been established that the patient has a bronchial carcinoma it is necessary to determine if the tumour is operable. In addition to the above, the following should be performed:

Haemoglobin, ESR, white blood count and film. If any of these are abnormal a bone marrow examination should be

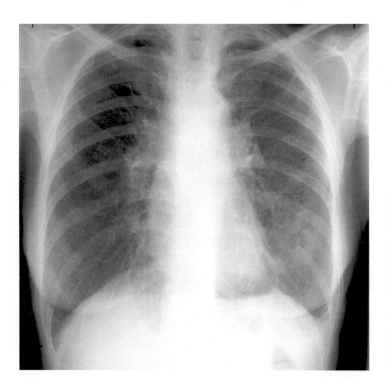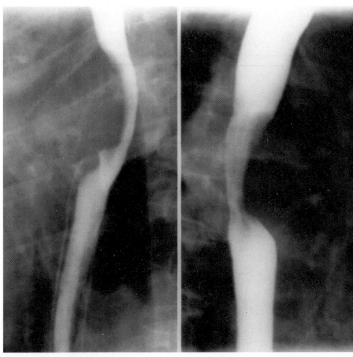

Fig. 3.39 Small cell carcinoma of the bronchus: bilateral hilar lymphadenopathy and widening of the mediastinum. A small left pleural effusion is present and there is widespread nodular shadowing in both lung fields. The patient presented with dysphagia. Barium swallow (right) shows compression and marked narrowing of the oesophagus by enlarged lymph nodes.

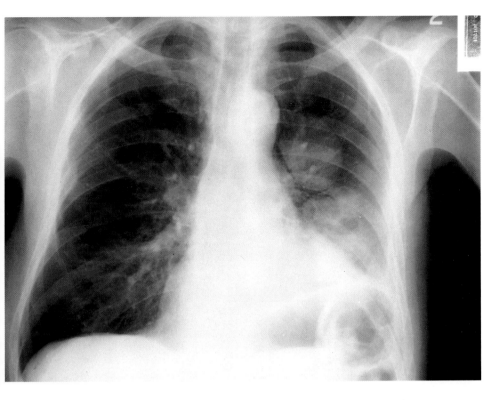

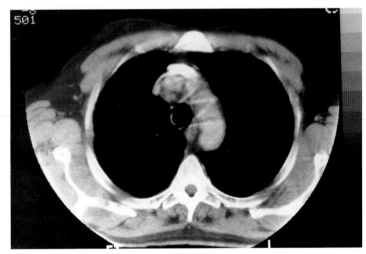

Fig. 3.40 Small cell carcinoma: a cavitating mass in the left lower lobe. A small left pleural effusion is present and the left dome of the diaphragm is elevated due to phrenic nerve involvement. An oval opacity above the carcinoma has well defined inferior margins and poorly defined upper margins. This is due to a loculated effusion in the oblique fissure. There are pathological fractures of several ribs on the right due to metastases.

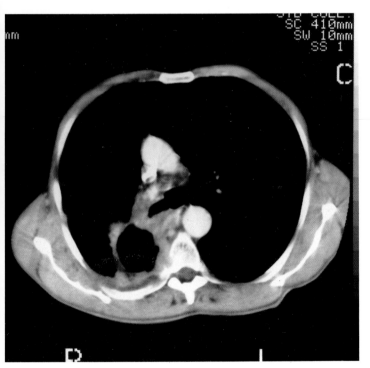

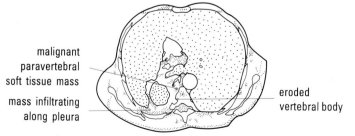

malignant paravertebral soft tissue mass

mass infiltrating along pleura

eroded vertebral body

Fig. 3.41 CT scan showing carcinoma involving vertebrae. Malignant infiltrates are seen in the right paravertebral gutter with destruction of the right posterior parts of the vertebrae.

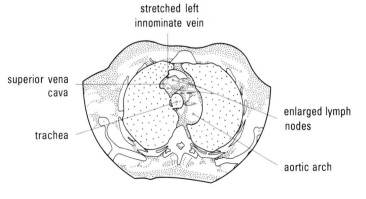

stretched left innominate vein

superior vena cava

trachea

enlarged lymph nodes

aortic arch

Fig. 3.42 CT scan showing enlarged lymph nodes between the arch of the aorta and the superior vena cava. The left innominate vein is stretched over the lymph nodes anteriorly.

performed. This should be performed in all cases of small cell carcinoma which frequently metastasizes to the bone marrow.

ECG. Most patients with bronchial carcinoma tend to be elderly and before embarking on a thoracotomy it is important to check on the state of the heart.

Urea, electrolytes and blood sugar.

Pulmonary function tests. Many patients with bronchial carcinoma have been heavy smokers and have bronchitis. If the lung function is poor, lobectomy or pneumonectomy may not be possible.

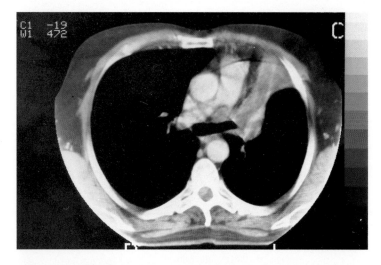

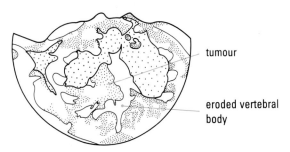

Fig. 3.43 CT scan showing collapse of the left upper lobe. Tumour is seen extending into the mediastinum in front of the bronchus and causing compression of the right pulmonary artery at its origin from the pulmonary trunk. The tumour has occluded the upper left lobe bronchus.

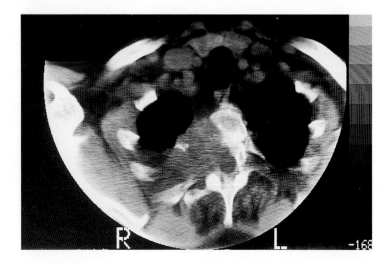

Fig. 3.44 CT scan of chest: Pancoast's tumour destroying part of the right side of the vertebrae and posterior ends of adjacent ribs.

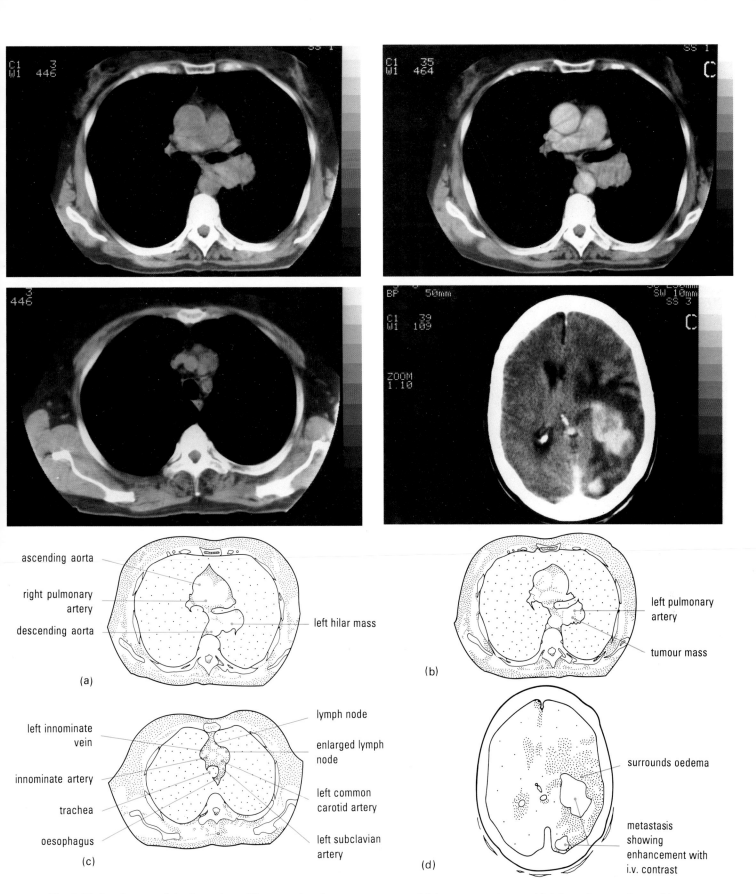

Fig. 3.45 Carcinoma of the bronchus. CT scans showing: (a) Primary mass in the left hilum surrounds the left pulmonary artery. (b) Following contrast enhancement the left pulmonary artery is seen to be considerably compressed by the mass. (c) Shows enlargement of nodes in the left superior mediastinum in front of the left common carotid artery. (d) Large metastases which have been enhanced by i.v. contrast medium and a smaller lesion posteriorly in the right cerebral hemisphere. There is considerable oedema around the lesion.

Bone scan. This is important if the patient has any symptoms suggestive of bony metastases, in which case thoracotomy would be inappropriate (Fig. 3.46). Some centres perform bone scans routinely in patients with bronchial carcinoma.

Liver scan. Patients with abnormalities in liver function tests or a palpable liver should have the liver investigated by scanning techniques and, if necessary, by liver biopsy (Fig. 3.47).

Isotope or CT scan of the brain. If the patient has any neurological symptoms or signs these scans should be performed. They should be performed in all cases of small cell tumour (Fig. 3.48; see also Fig. 3.45).

Differential diagnosis

The differential diagnosis includes all causes of a solitary pulmonary nodule and, in addition, recurrent pneumonia, tuberculosis and pulmonary infarction.

Prognosis

This is very poor but squamous cell carcinoma has a better prognosis than carcinoma of other cell types. Tumours are staged by size, position and extent of lymph node and other organ involvement using the TNM staging system (Fig. 3.49). The more limited tumours have the better prognosis. Surgery is the only treatment which offers a chance of cure but only about twenty-five percent of patients are suitable for surgery at

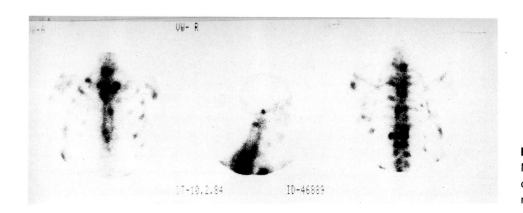

Fig. 3.46 Skeletal metastases. Multiple areas of increased uptake of the radio-isotope ^{99m}Tc indicate metastases.

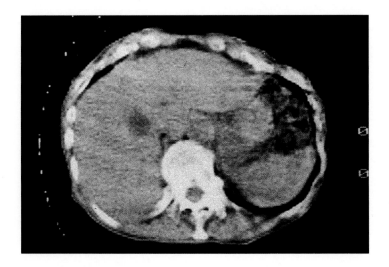

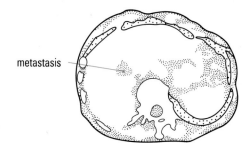

metastasis

Fig. 3.47 CT scan of liver: areas of decreased enhancement representing metastases are seen in the right lobe of the liver.

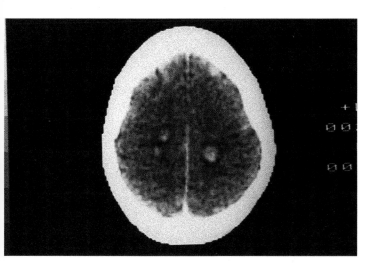

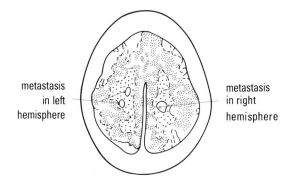
metastasis
in left
hemisphere

metastasis
in right
hemisphere

Fig. 3.48 CT scan showing cerebral metastases. Multiple contrast-enhanced lesions are seen in both cerebral hemispheres.

TNM staging system for carcinoma of the bronchus

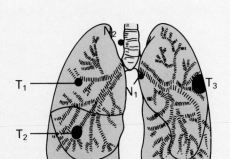

STAGE GROUPINGS OF TNM SUBSETS

Occult carcinoma	TX	N0	M0
Stage 0	TIS	Carcinoma in situ	
Stage I	T1	N0	M0
	T2	N0	M0
Stage II	T1	N1	M0
	T2	N1	M0
Stage IIIa	T3	N0	M0
	T3	N1	M0
	T1–3	N2	M0
Stage IIIb	Any T	N3	M0
	T4	Any N	M0
Stage IV	Any T	Any N	M1

TNM DEFINITIONS

Primary Tumour

TX   Tumour proven by the presence of malignant cells in bronchopulmonary secretions but not visualized roentgenographically or bronchoscopically, or any tumour that cannot be assessed as in a retreatment staging.

TO   No evidence of primary tumour.

TIS   Carcinoma *in situ*.

T1   A tumour that is 3.0cm or less in greatest dimension, surrounded by lung or visceral pleura, and without evidence of invasion proximal to a lobar bronchus at bronchoscopy.

T2   A tumour more than 3.0cm in greatest dimension, or a tumour of any size that either invades the visceral pleura or has associated atelectasis or obstructive pneumonitis extending to the hilar region. At bronchoscopy, the proximal extent of demonstrable tumour must be within a lobar bronchus or at least 2.0cm distal to the carina. Any associated atelectasis or obstructive pneumonitis must involve less than an entire lung.

T3   A tumour of any size with direct extension into the chest wall (including superior sulcus tumours), diaphragm, or the mediastinal pleura or pericardium without involving the heart, great vessels, trachea, oesophagus or vertebral body, or a tumour in the main bronchus within 2cm of the carina without involving the carina.

T4   A tumour of any size with invasion of the mediastinum or involving heart, great vessels, trachea, oesophagus, vertebral body or carina or presence of malignant pleural effusion.

Nodal Involvement (N)

N0   No demonstrable metastasis to regional lymph nodes.

N1   Metastasis to lymph nodes in the peribronchial or the ipsilateral hilar region, or both, including direct extension.

N2   Metastasis to ipsilateral mediastinal lymph nodes and subcarinal lymph nodes.

N3   Metastasis to contralateral mediastinal lymph nodes, contralateral hilar lymph nodes, ipsilateral or contralateral scalene or supraclavicular lymph nodes.

Distant Metastasis (M)

M0   No (known) distant metastasis.

M1   Distant metastasis present — specify site(s).

Fig. 3.49 TNM staging system for carcinoma of the bronchus.

the time of presentation. The five-year survival after surgery is only about thirty percent. This is due to recurrence from micrometastases which were undetected at the time of surgery (Fig. 3.50). Overall, less than ten percent of patients survive five years.

Treatment

Surgery

This involves lobectomy or pneumonectomy depending on the extent of the tumour (Fig. 3.51). This should only be carried out if extensive investigation has excluded metastases as far as is possible.

Contraindications to surgery include:

Advanced age, as survival after pneumonectomy is not good over the age of 70.

Inadequate lung function. Surgery is contraindicated if the FEV_1 is less than 1 litre or if the arterial carbon dioxide is raised. This excludes many patients who have coexisting chronic bronchitis.

Local extension of tumour into the lymph nodes, recurrent laryngeal nerve, phrenic nerve, pleura or superior vena cava.

Distant metastases to the brain, bone, liver or other sites.

Significant disease in any other system, e.g. recent myocardial infarction, poor cardiac function or renal failure.

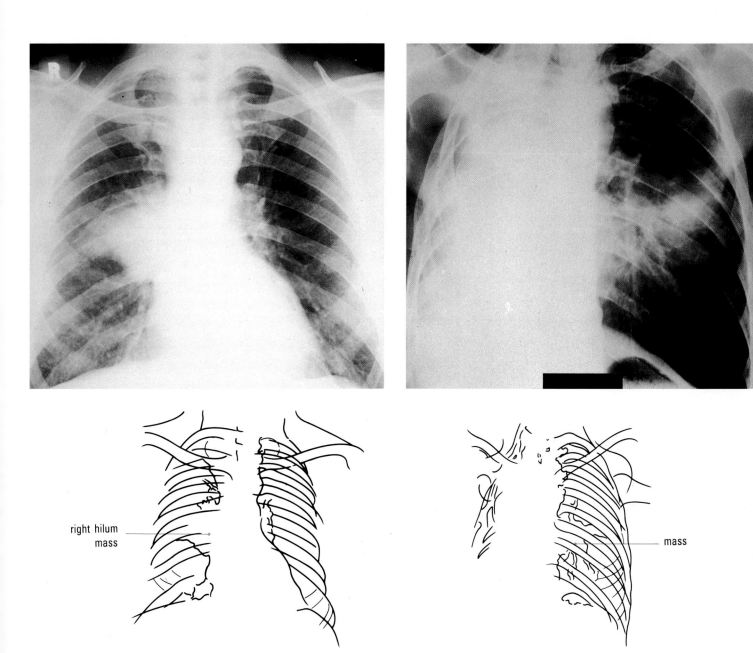

Fig. 3.50 Mass at the right hilum: squamous cell carcinoma treated by pneumonectomy. Eight years later (right) a mass is present in the left lung. This could be a fresh primary or a recurrence.

Radiotherapy

Radiotherapy is hardly ever curative in bronchial carcinoma but may produce some regression of the tumour (Fig. 3.52). Prolonged therapy can cause pneumonitis (Fig. 3.53). In most centres it is now considered inappropriate to give prolonged courses of radiotherapy as they do not prolong life. However, palliative radiotherapy is widely used as it gives symptomatic relief of superior vena cava obstruction, stridor, haemoptysis, bone pain, dysphagia and cerebral secondaries. Often a short course of radiotherapy which produces no side effects but gives marked relief of symptoms can be given.

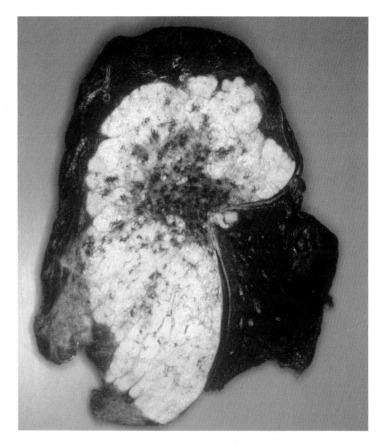

Fig. 3.51 A pneumonectomy specimen in which the lung is largely replaced by carcinoma.

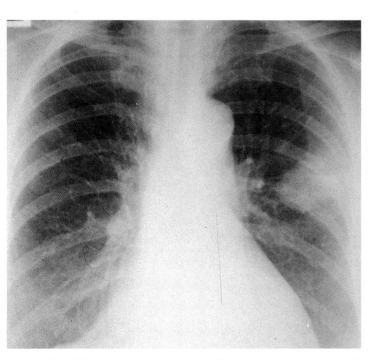 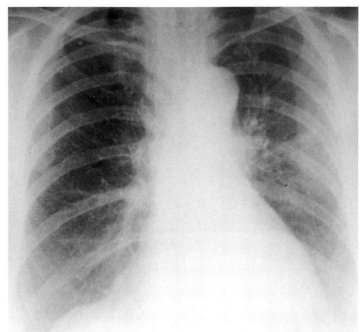

Fig. 3.52 Anaplastic carcinoma. Mass in the left mid zone. Following radiotherapy (right) the mass is smaller and only a small shadow persists in the left mid zone.

Chemotherapy

There is undoubted evidence that small cell carcinoma is responsive to chemotherapy (Figs 3.54 and 3.55). Many regimens involving multiple drugs are currently being tested. These prolong life but very rarely effect a cure. There is a price to pay in that most chemotherapeutic drugs have side effects such as alopecia, neutropenia, thrombocytopenia, anaemia, nausea, vomiting or peripheral neuropathy. Great care has to be given in the administration of these drugs as some may cause necrosis if injected outside a vein in error (Fig. 3.56). There is, as yet,

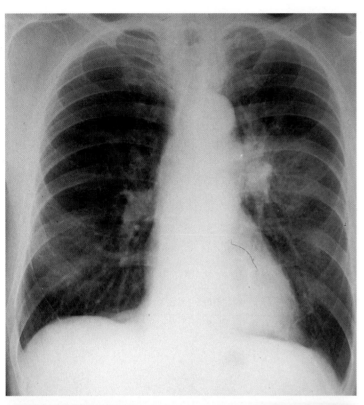

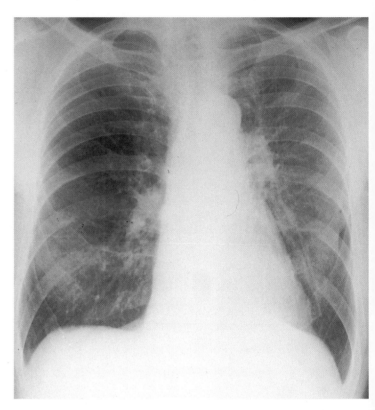

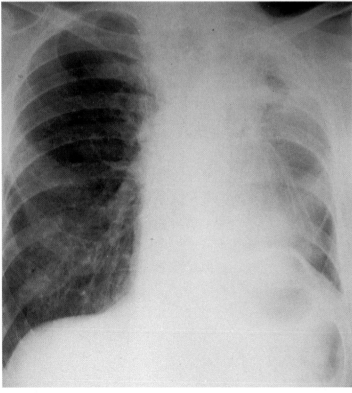

Fig. 3.53 (a) Carcinoma adjacent to the left hilum: large cell tumour. (b) Post-radiation pneumonitis following prolonged therapy leading to (c) fibrosis and collapse of the left upper lobe.

little evidence that chemotherapy should be used in tumours of the bronchus other than small cell carcinoma. Injections of chemotherapeutic agents such as mustine or bleomycin into the pleura may be used to prevent reaccumulation of malignant pleural effusions.

Immunotherapy

Attempts have been made to treat bronchial carcinoma with intrapleural BCG in conjunction with surgery, and *Corynebacterium parvum* in conjunction with chemotherapy. These attempts have not met with success and this form of treatment has been largely abandoned.

Symptomatic treatment

This is extremely important as the majority of patients are not suitable for surgery. It is important to consider the patient as a whole and give them plenty of time to talk about their condition, their fears and the treatment modalities which have been suggested to them. For many frail patients no treatment may be indicated initially. Surgery, radiotherapy or chemotherapy would only give distressing side effects with no increase in survival. However, the patient should be reassured that if he develops any troublesome symptoms then appropriate treatment will be given. As the disease progresses, radiotherapy may be indicated to palliate a specific symptom.

If a patient develops obstruction of the trachea or main bronchus, temporary symptomatic relief may be provided by use of a laser via the fibreoptic bronchoscope or implantation of radioactive gold grains or other local radiotherapy.

A patient may need codeine or morphine to suppress an irritating cough. Some patients benefit from bronchodilators. Simple analgesics may be required and sedatives may be used to relieve anxiety. Opiates should be used in adequate dosage to control symptoms such as pain and dyspnoea — the most appropriate is often morphine linctus given together with stemetil to control any nausea.

The physician should take care to work closely with the nursing staff, medical social workers, occupational therapists, physiotherapists, chaplain, general practitioner and district nurse to provide good symptom control, good nursing care, emotional, spiritual and social support for the patient and their family.

Prevention

The major aetiological factor is cigarette smoking and effort must therefore be undertaken to stop smoking using health education and prohibition of cigarette advertisement and smoking in public places. Much of this requires government action. However all health care workers have a responsibility, both by example and education, to inform the public of the dangers inherent in smoking.

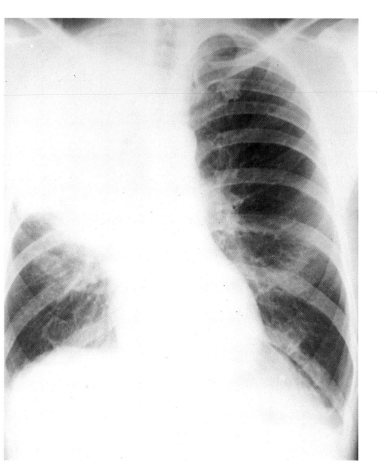 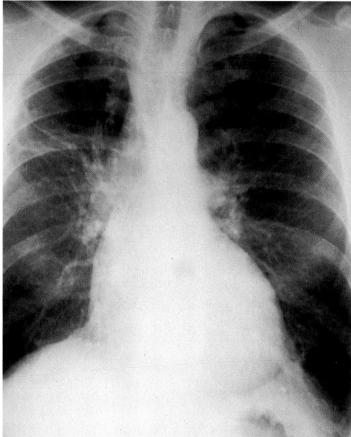

Fig. 3.54 Small cell carcinoma. Collapse and consolidation of the right upper lobe and a mass at the right hilum. Following treatment (right) there has been considerable improvement.

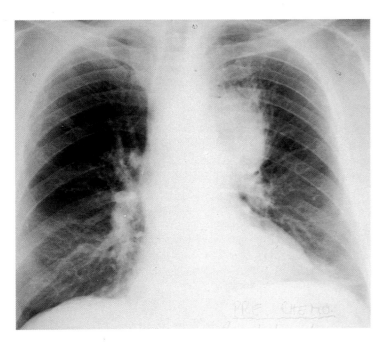
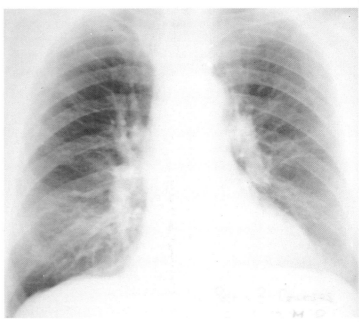

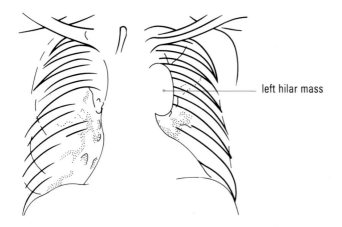

left hilar mass

Fig. 3.55 Small cell carcinoma. Frontal views showing left hilar mass before and (right) after chemotherapy.

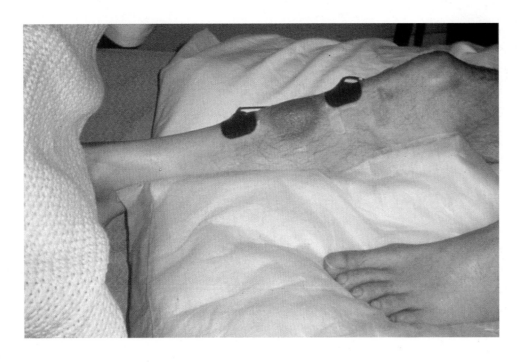

Fig. 3.56 The effects of chemotherapy inadvertently injected outside a vein.

OTHER TUMOURS OF THE LUNG

Alveolar cell carcinoma (bronchiolo-alveolar cell carcinoma)

Alveolar cell carcinoma arises from the bronchiolo-alveolar epithelium (Figs 3.57 and 3.58). Its incidence is about 100 times less common than bronchial carcinoma. It characteristically grows along the alveolar walls and is liable to be multifocal in one or both lungs. It comprises 1.5% of all malignant tumours of the lung. Patients may be asymptomatic or they may present with copious amounts of watery sputum, cough or haemoptysis. As the disease progresses patients may become very breathless and show systemic symptoms of malignancy.

Death is usually from respiratory failure. The chest radiograph will show solitary or multiple shadows which are often bilateral. Malignant cells may be found in the sputum but bronchoscopy is usually unhelpful. Transbronchial biopsy, percutaneous lung biopsy or open surgical resection may be necessary to establish a diagnosis. The differential diagnosis includes bronchial carcinoma, tuberculosis and pneumonia. Surgical treatment offers a chance of cure if the tumour is localized, but the tumour is relatively resistant to chemotherapy and radiotherapy. Survival is better than for bronchial carcinoma, especially if the disease is localized. Patients with multifocal disease often die quickly, but in a few patients the survival may be fairly long even without specific treatment.

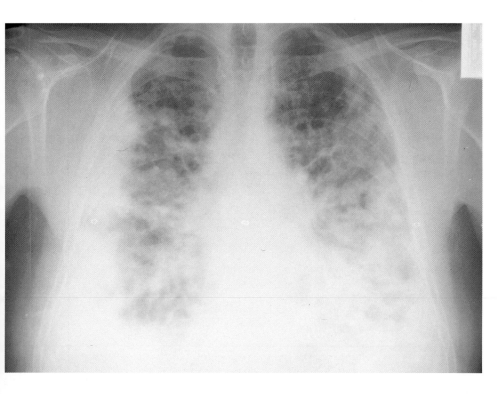

Fig. 3.57 Bronchiolo-alveolar cell carcinoma: widespread poorly defined nodular shadowing which is confluent over a large area in both lungs, particularly peripherally.

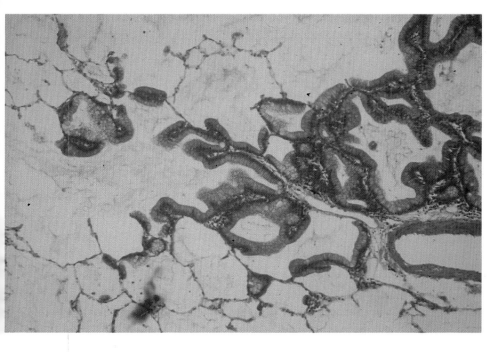

Fig. 3.58 Histology, bronchiolo-alveolar cell carcinoma. Rather than destroying the lung substance, the tumour cells are growing along the alveolar walls, using them as a scaffold. Bronchiolo-alveolar carcinoma is a primary lung tumour that has this growth pattern throughout its substance. This pattern of growth is often seen at the margins of an ordinary adenocarcinoma and may also be seen in adenocarcinomas of other organs that metastasize to the lung. Histology cannot distinguish between these tumour types.

Pulmonary lymphomas

These arise from lymphoid tissue within the lung and typically remain localized for considerable periods of time. They may be Hodgkin's or non-Hodgkin's lymphomas and presentation may be similar to other types of pulmonary tumour (Fig. 3.59). The radiological appearance includes glandular enlargement, pulmonary infiltrates, disseminated nodules, coin lesions, or unilateral hilar masses resembling carcinoma of the bronchus. Pleural effusions may also be present. Treatment is by chemotherapy and/or radiotherapy, as for other lymphomas. The pulmonary lesion has however usually to be removed to make the diagnosis.

Melanoma of the bronchus

This is a rare tumour. It is probably derived from the embryonic melanoblasts incorporated in the laryngotracheal bud. It is very difficult to exclude a metastasis from a forgotten skin primary lesion.

Sarcomas

Sarcomas of the lung are rare. Local invasion and metastases may occur but tumour often remains localized. Lymphosarcoma, leiomyosarcoma, rhabdomyosarcoma, chondrosarcoma, neurosarcoma, fibrosarcoma, osteosarcoma and haemangiopericytoma have all been reported.

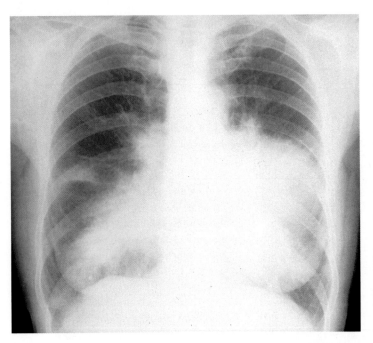
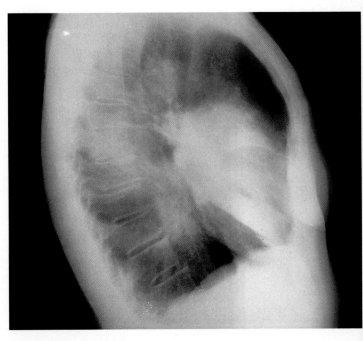

Fig. 3.59 Lymphocytic lymphoma of the lung. Ill-defined areas of dense opacification are present in both lungs; similarly areas of consolidation. These developed slowly over several years.

Carcinosarcoma

These tumours of malignant epithelial and malignant stroma are rare. They are more common in men and present similarly to bronchial carcinoma occluding the bronchial lumen.

Pulmonary blastoma

This is derived from undifferentiated embryonic connective tissue (Fig. 3.60) and is another very rare tumour which sometimes has a benign course but may metastasize.

Carcinoids

This is the commonest of the bronchial adenomas and may present as a polyp (Fig. 3.61) in the bronchus. A bronchial carcinoid tumour (Figs 3.62–3.64) may give rise to the carcinoid syndrome which consists of intermittent cyanotic flushes,

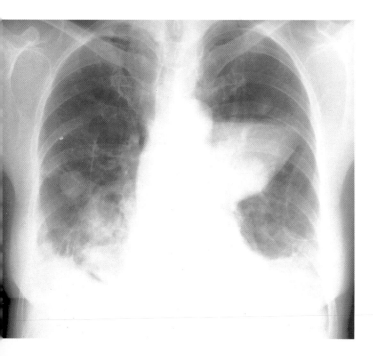

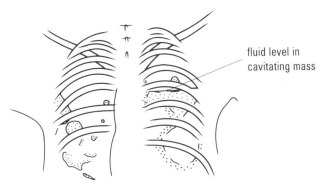

Fig. 3.60 Pulmonary blastoma: multiple round opacities some of which have cavitated (an air fluid level is seen opposite the aortic knuckle in one large lesion).

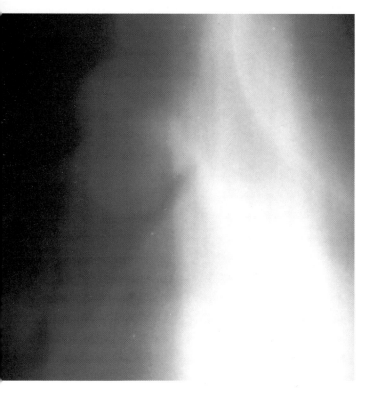

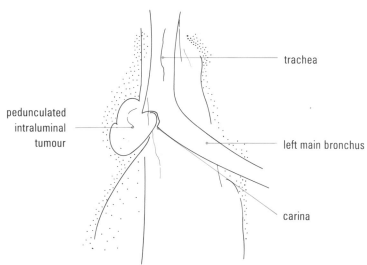

Fig. 3.61 Bronchial carcinoid tumour. The tomogram shows a pedunculated intraluminal tumour at the origin of the right main bronchus.

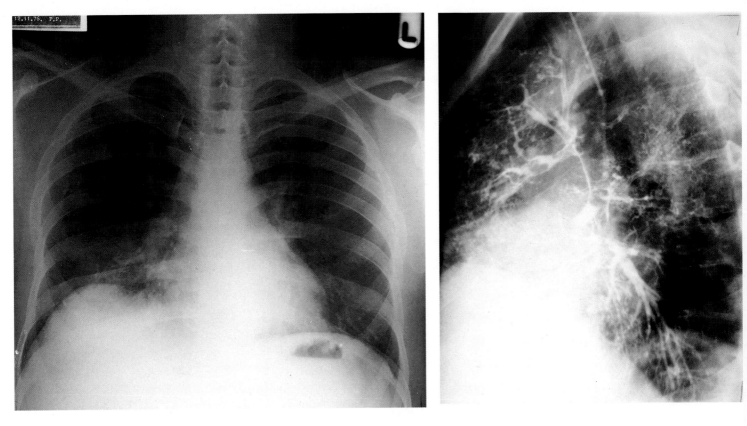

Fig. 3.62 Carcinoid tumour of the right middle lobe bronchus. There is shadowing adjacent to the right heart border which is obscured due to collapse of the right middle lobe. In the bronchogram (right) the middle lobe bronchus is totally occluded 1cm from its origin. The bronchus does not narrow like a rat tail as it would with a more malignant tumour.

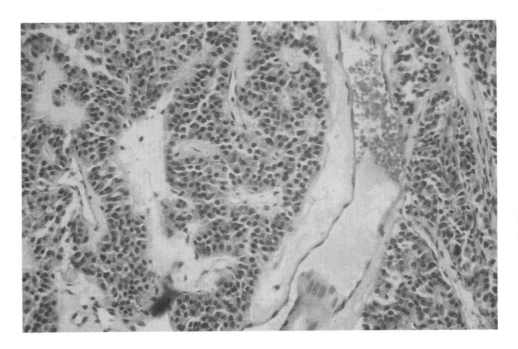

Fig. 3.63 Histology, carcinoid tumour. The tumour cells are arranged in cords (trabecular pattern) and regular in appearance, lacking the atypia that characterizes more malignant tumours.

abdominal cramps, diarrhoea, wheezing and dyspnoea. These symptoms are thought to be due to the production of serotonin and kinins. Breakdown products of serotonin can be identified in the urine. Most patients with carcinoid symptoms have metastases (Fig. 3.65), usually in the liver, in which case valvular disease affecting the right heart may develop. The chest radiograph may be abnormal, but it is often normal and diagnosis is made following bronchoscopy and biopsy. If the tumour can be resected the prognisis is good and even patients with metastases may have a reasonable survival.

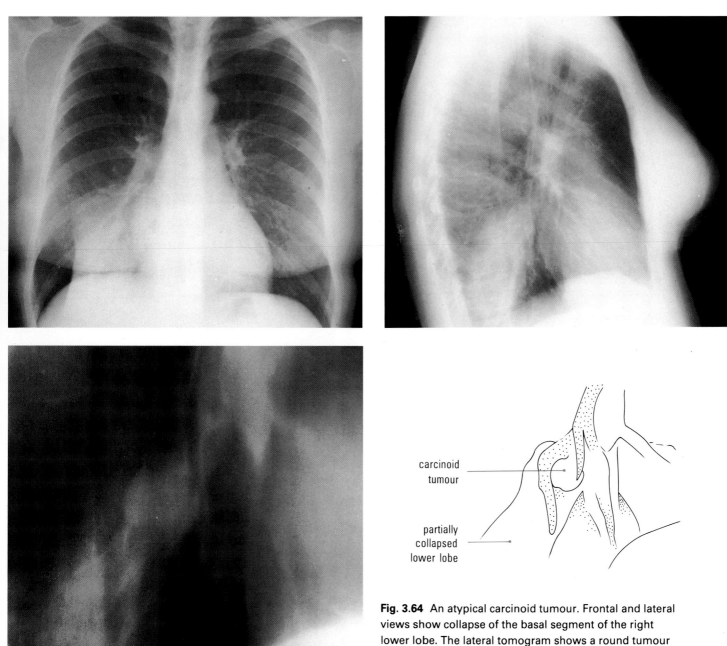

carcinoid tumour

partially collapsed lower lobe

Fig. 3.64 An atypical carcinoid tumour. Frontal and lateral views show collapse of the basal segment of the right lower lobe. The lateral tomogram shows a round tumour compressing and narrowing the lower lobe bronchus.

Bronchial gland tumours

Adenocystic carcinoma (cylindroma) (Figs 3.66 and 3.67), mucoepidermoid carcinoma and mixed tumours all arise from the bronchial mucous glands, often in the large bronchi, whose

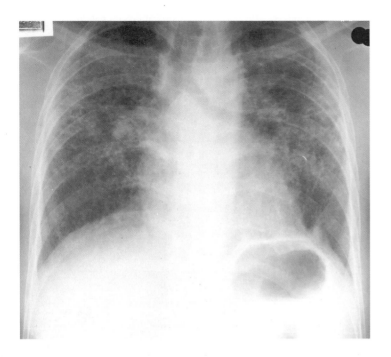

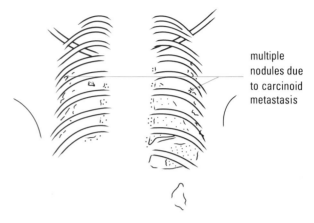

Fig. 3.65 Bronchial carcinoid tumour with diffuse pulmonary involvement. Nodular shadowing in both lungs due to metastases from a carcinoid which originated at the right hilum.

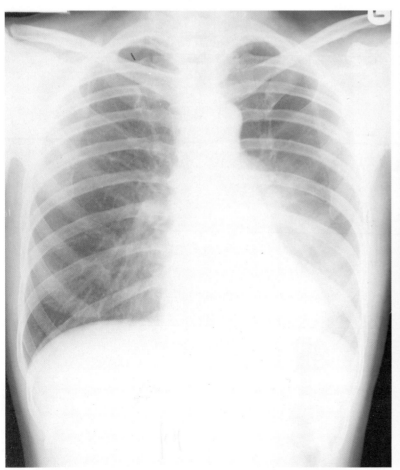

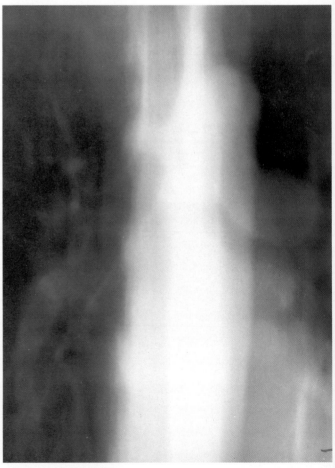

Fig. 3.66 Adenoid cystic carcinoma (cylindroma). The mass at the left hilum is due to nodal involvement. There is some consolidation of the left lower lobe. Tomogram shows a tumour almost totally occluding the left main bronchus at its origin.

wall they infiltrate. Rarely the tumour may be a benign mucous gland adenoma or cystadenoma (Fig. 3.68). They may present with recurrent haemoptysis, cough, unilateral wheezing, pulmonary collapse and infection. Patients tend to be younger

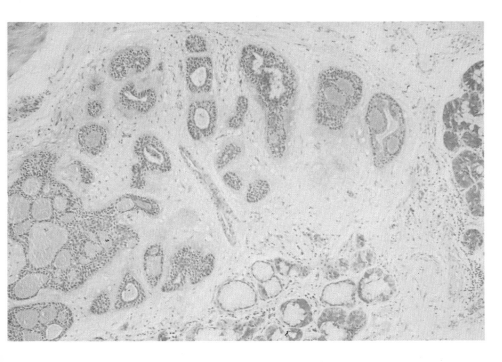

Fig. 3.67 Adenoid cystic carcinoma (cylindroma) histology.

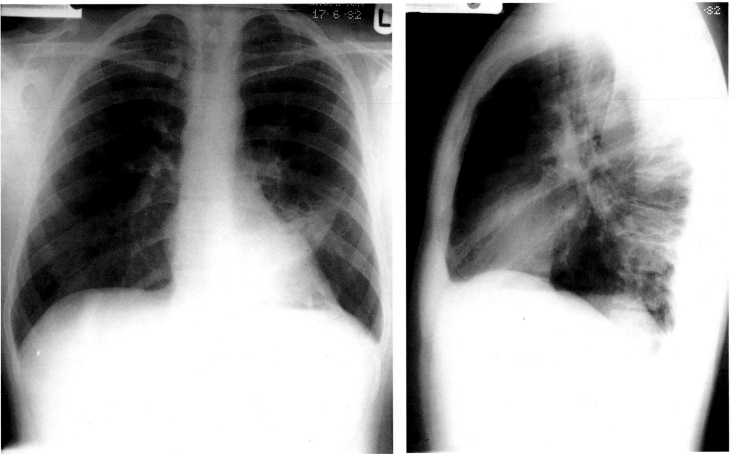

Fig. 3.68 Mucous gland adenoma of the bronchus. Frontal and lateral views showing area of collapse adjacent to the posterior basal segment of the left lower lobe. Bronchoscopy (not shown) revealed tumour in the left lower lobe bronchus distal to the apical lower bronchus.

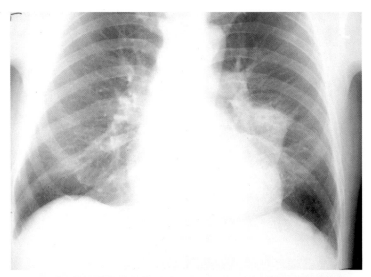

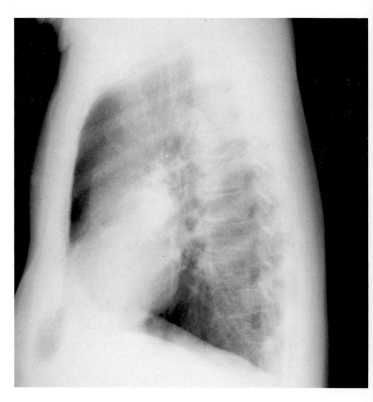

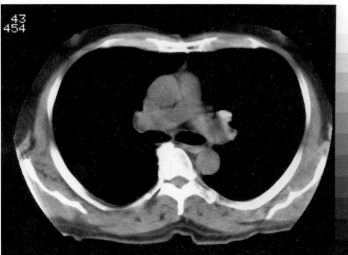

Fig. 3.69 Hamartoma. Frontal and lateral views show collapse of the lingula. CT scan shows tumour of the left hilum with calcification within it.

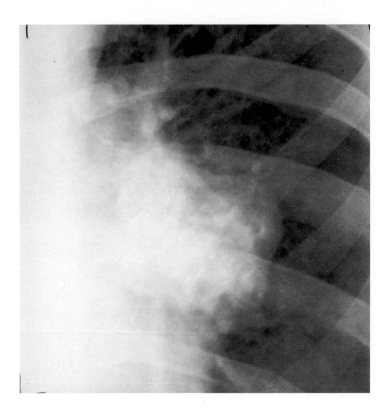

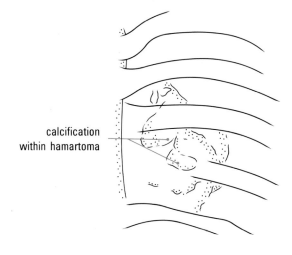

calcification within hamartoma

Fig. 3.70 Hamartoma showing typical calcification.

than those with carcinoma of the bronchus. These tumours may metastasize but many of the tumours grow slowly.

Hamartoma

This tumour is composed of different tissues which normally appear in the lung but they are abnormally organized to form a tumour (Figs 3.69–3.71). The lesion usually arises in the periphery of the lung and may be found on a routine chest X-ray, and usually occurs after the age of fifty years. Hamartoma should be considered in the differential diagnosis of any coin lesion on chest radiograph. Treatment is by surgical resection.

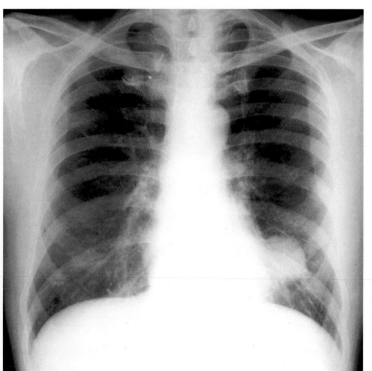

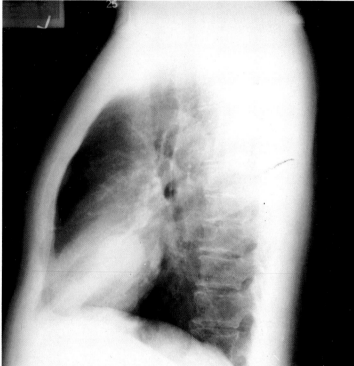

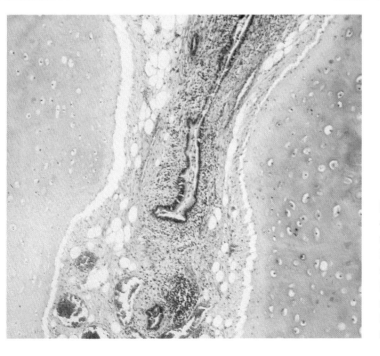

Fig. 3.71 Hamartoma. Frontal and lateral views show a 4cm mass present in the lingula. No calcification is seen within it to indicate its benign nature. Histology shows a bizarre mixture of mature cartilage and respiratory epithelium which led to the view that these lesions were hamartomatous but many believe that the epithelial clefts are merely entrapped air spaces and that the increasing incidence with age favours a neoplastic rather than developmental aetiology.

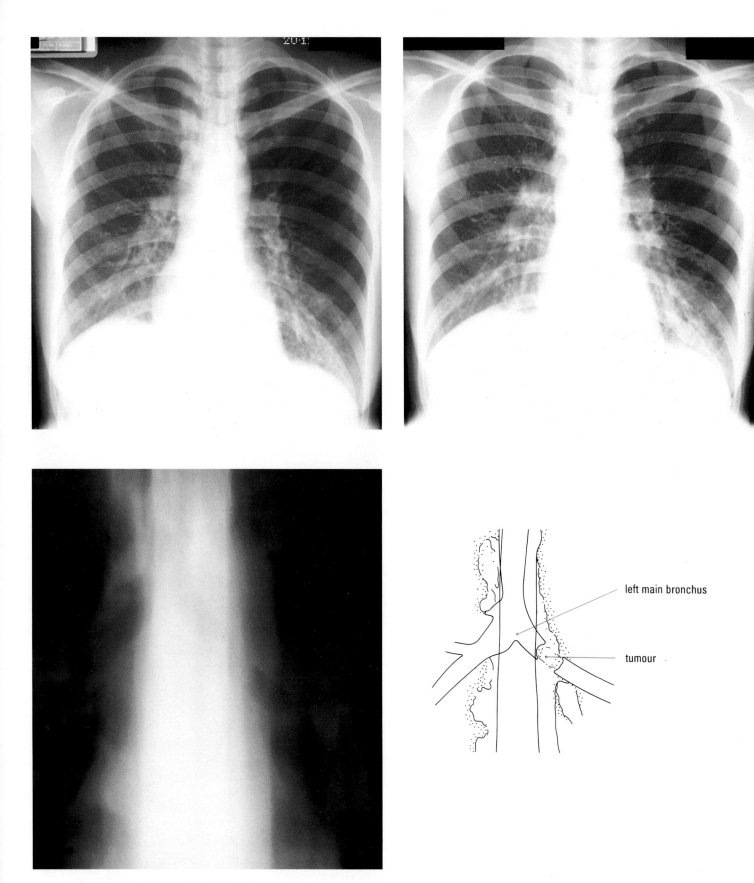

left main bronchus

tumour

Fig. 3.72 Papilloma of the left main bronchus. Expiratory film (upper left) shows there is air trapping in the left lung and the left dome of the diaphragm does not move. The mediastinum shifts to the right on expiration. Inspiratory film (upper right). In this frontal view inflammatory changes at the left base are seen. Tomogram (lower) shows tumour of the left main bronchus (an anomalous bronchus rises from the right main bronchus).

Papilloma

Papillomata of trachea or bronchus are rare and usually occur in young people (Fig. 3.72). This tumour consists of a connective tissue core covered by squamous epithelium.

Plasma cell granuloma

This lesion consists of plasma cells, spindle cells, lymphocytes and blood vessels. Haemoptysis is a frequent presenting symptom. The lesion is usually within the lung substance and may involve the bronchus (Fig. 3.73).

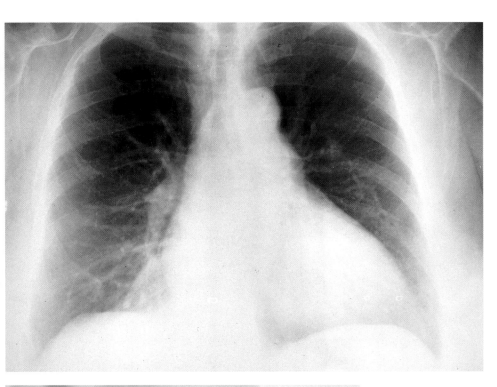

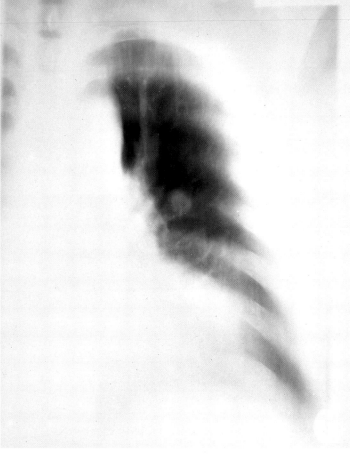

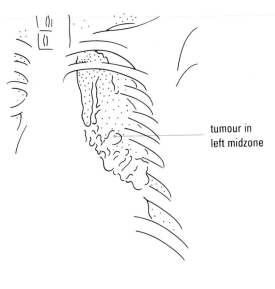

tumour in left midzone

Fig. 3.73 Plasma cell granuloma: frontal view and tomogram show the clearly defined tumour in the left middle zone. There are no specific radiological features.

Pulmonary metastases

The common sites of a primary tumour which metastasizes to the lungs are breast, pancreas, stomach, skin, kidney, ovary, prostate, uterus (Figs 3.74 and 3.75), thyroid (Fig. 3.76) and testes (Fig. 3.77).

Pulmonary metastasis may cause the following radiographic appearances: extensive lesions (Fig. 3.78), solitary pulmonary nodules (Fig. 3.79), multiple nodules (Fig. 3.80) or lymphangitis carcinomatosa (see Fig. 3.15). Many pulmonary metastases do not cause any symptoms but breathlessness may occur with the development of lymphangitis carcinomatosa. Pleural effusions may form due to secondary malignant deposits in the pleura.

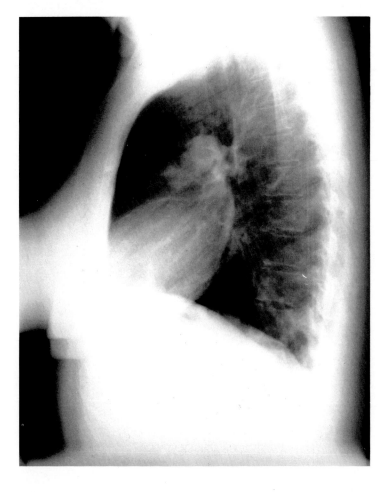

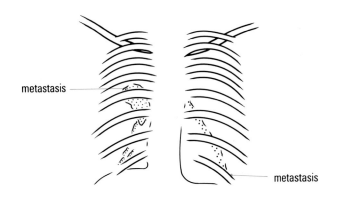

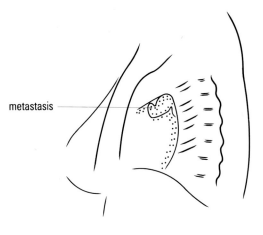

Fig. 3.74 Metastatic 'leiomyoma'. The patient had a hysterectomy for fibroids 7 years previously. Clearly defined round opacities are present in front and to the right of the right hilum. Another is seen in the left costophrenic angle.

The solitary round nodule in the lung

Frequently a circumscribed opacity in the lung is a chance finding on a routine radiograph and poses a diagnostic problem. The approach to diagnosis should begin with establishing, if possible, how long the lesion has been present. If calcification is present within the lesion it is almost certainly benign, except for the occasional carcinoma developing in association with an old tuberculous focus or other calcified granuloma. It may be necessary to perform tomography to demonstrate calcification or to show abnormal feeding vessels in arteriovenous fistula but, in most instances, with good-quality, high-kilovoltage radiographs, tomography nowadays adds little or no useful additional information. Rather, an attempt at obtaining a histological or cytological diagnosis should be made. Sputum should be examined; if negative, fibreoptic bronchoscopy, with washing and brushings, and transbronchial biopsy may be under-

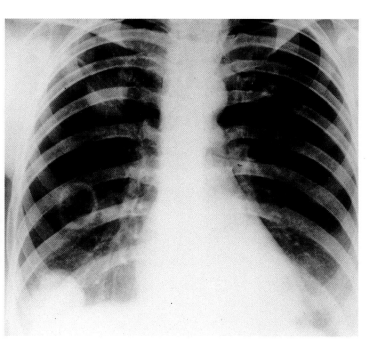

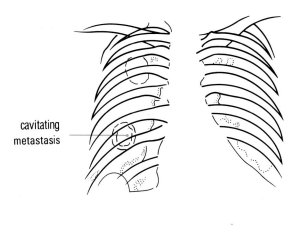

Fig. 3.75 Cavitating metastases from carcinoma of the cervix.

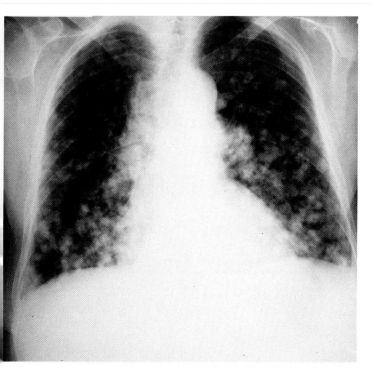

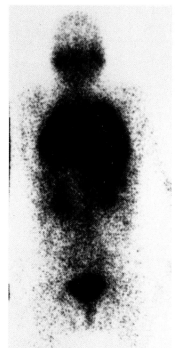

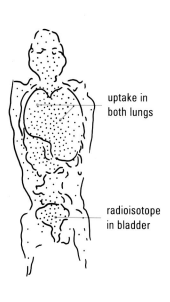

Fig. 3.76 Metastases from a follicular cell carcinoma of the thyroid. Frontal view shows multiple round opacities in both lungs with lymphadenopathy at the right hilum and right paratracheal region. Radioiodine scan of the lungs shows uptake in both lungs.

taken. Recourse to direct percutaneous aspiration needle biopsy under fluoroscopic or CT control (Fig. 3.81) may be necessary if results so far have been unrewarding. Finally, it may be necessary to perform a thoracotomy and open biopsy to establish a diagnosis. The general clinical picture, including the age of the patient and the smoking history, will obviously influence the degree to which investigation is pursued.

The use of CT in the diagnosis of the solitary pulmonary nodule has in recent years received impetus following reports from a few centres that the density of the lesion indicates whether it is benign or malignant. Many benign lesions are more dense, with a higher CT number, than malignant lesions; this is probably because of microscopic amounts of calcification present within them.

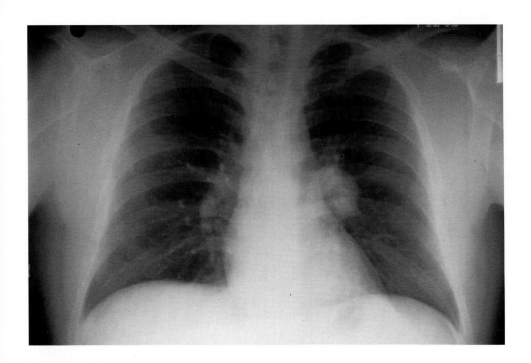

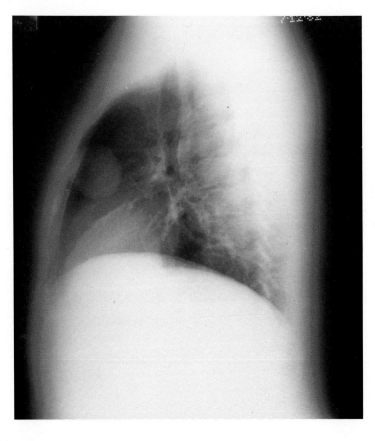

Fig. 3.77 Metastases from a testicular tumour three years after orchidectomy, frontal and lateral views show a clearly defined mass in the anterior segment of the left upper lobe.

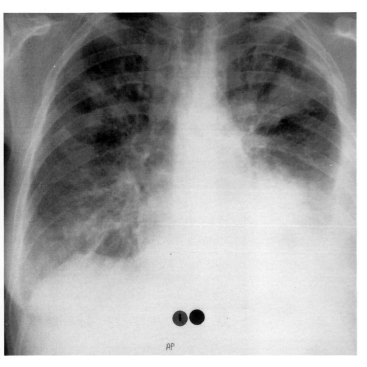

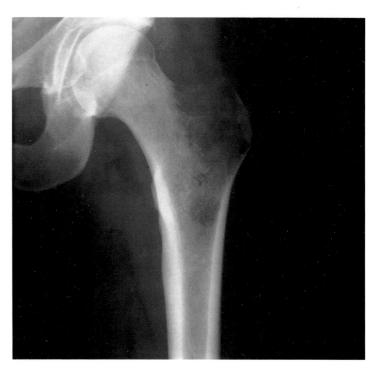

Fig. 3.78 Carcinoma of the breast with extensive pulmonary and bone metastases. Frontal view shows that a left mastectomy has been performed. There is a left pleural effusion and diffuse nodular shadowing confluent in places. Linear shadowing is present in both lungs due to extensive intrapulmonary spread. The left 4th rib is destroyed in the axilla by metastases. Left hip metastases (right) causing destruction of the greater trochanter.

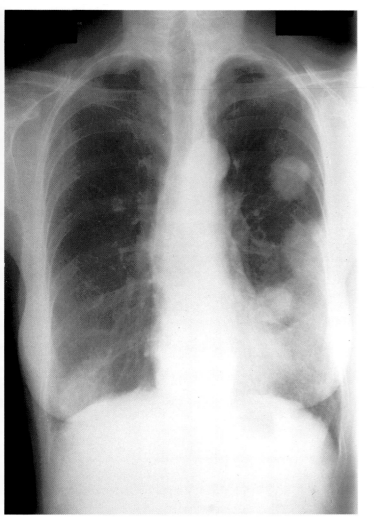

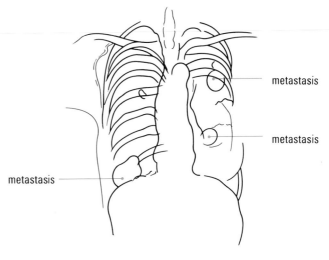

Fig. 3.79 Frontal view shows large, left-sided opacities due to metastases from an unknown primary.

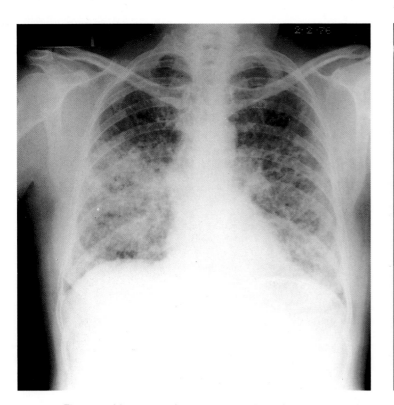
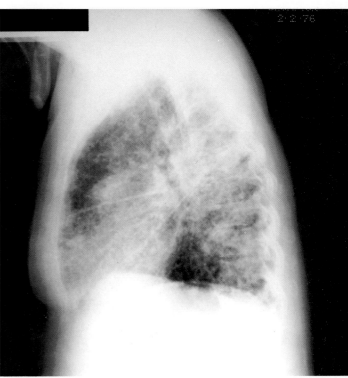

Fig. 3.80 Metastases from a primary bronchial adenocarcinoma. Frontal and lateral views show widespread small nodules throughout both lungs.

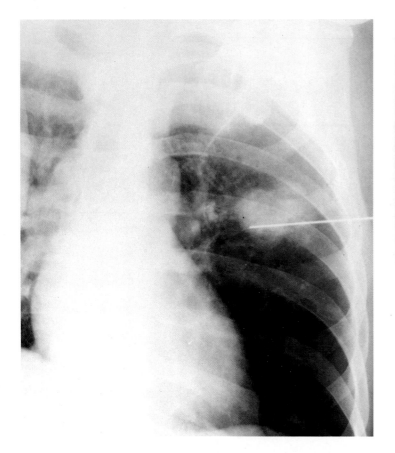

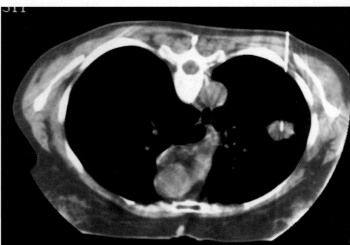

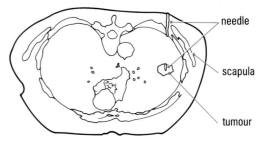

Fig. 3.81 Carcinoma. The radiograph was taken during aspiration needle biopsy under fluoroscopic control and shows the tip of the needle in a nodule in the lung. Histology revealed a squamous cell carcinoma. The CT scan shows a needle in a carcinoma of the left lung during biopsy under CT control. The needle can be seen in the soft tissues, with its tip in the lesion; the portion between is not visible on this window setting.

PLEURAL TUMOURS

Benign tumours

Benign cysts of the pleura (Fig. 3.82) and pleural tumours are rare and often asymptomatic. Finger clubbing, hypertrophic pulmonary osteoarthropathy and some chest pain are all possible presentations in pleural fibroma (Fig. 3.83). Surgical removal (Figs 3.84 and 3.85) is indicated to exclude malignancy.

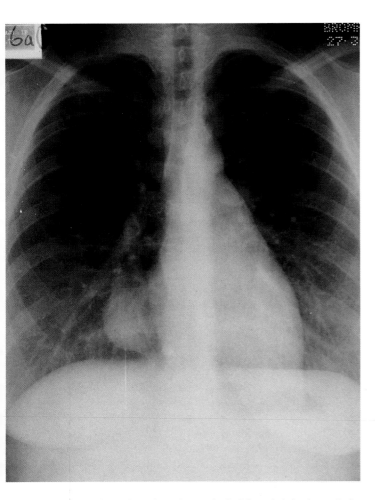 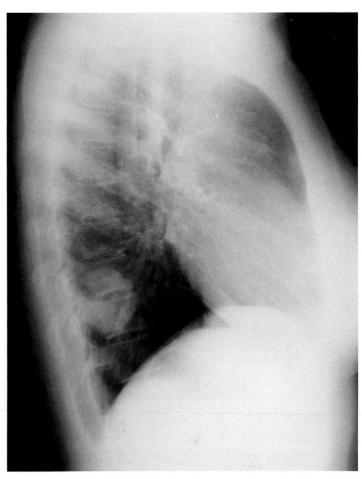

Fig. 3.82 A benign pleural cyst. Left, PA and right, lateral views.

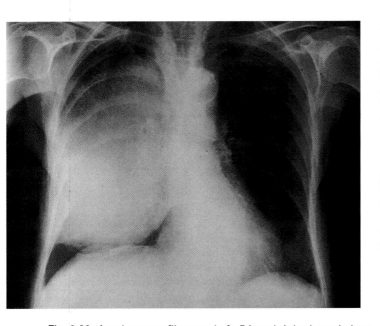 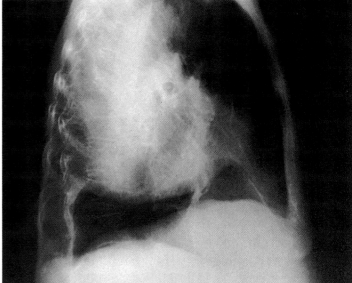

Fig. 3.83 A pulmonary fibroma. Left, PA and right, lateral views.

Malignant mesothelioma

In most patients malignant mesothelioma (Fig. 3.86) is associated with a history of asbestos inhalation, generally many years previously. Histologically the tumours may be of sarcomatous (Figs 3.87 and 3.88 left), epithelial (Figs 3.88 middle and 3.89) or mixed (Fig. 3.88 right) type. The patient may present with

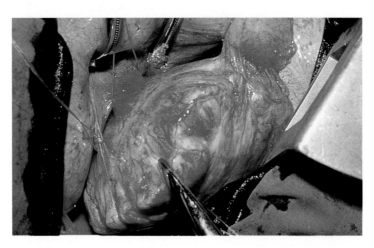

Fig. 3.84 Pleural fibroma, appearance at surgery. The appearances are those of a well demarcated tumour with lobulated but otherwise smooth surface.

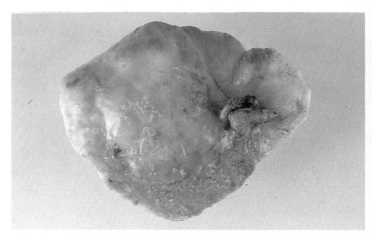

Fig. 3.85 Pleural fibroma excised. The specimen shows a smooth lobulated external surface with a pedicle forming a small tag.

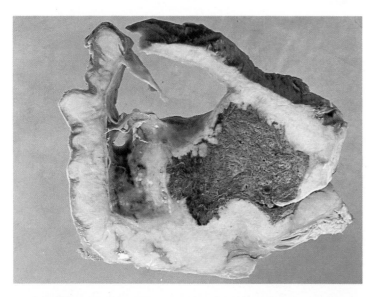

Fig. 3.86 Mesothelioma. A thick layer of pale tumour tissue surrounds the lung and forms a cavity which was originally filled with mucoid material.

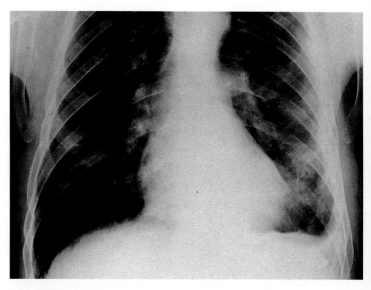

Fig. 3.87 Sarcomatous mesothelioma. Pleural shadowing with nodulation behind the heart, in the left costophrenic angle and along the lateral chest wall is seen. There is partial destruction by the tumour of the left 7th and 8th ribs in the axillar.

chest pain, pleurisy or dyspnoea due to a large pleural effusion (Fig. 3.90). The diagnosis is usually made following a pleural biopsy or thoracotomy. Pleural effusions should be controlled if necessary by pleurectomy and adequate analgesia given. Treatment is very unsatisfactory; most patients die within two years.

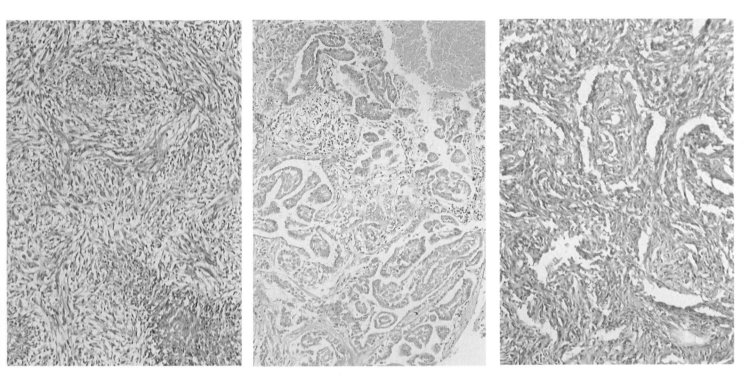

Fig. 3.88 Malignant mesothelioma. Left, sarcomatous type. The tumour consists of interweaving bundles of spindle cells. Haematoxylin and eosin stain. Middle, epithelial cell type. The tumour consists of adenopapillary structures. There is an area of necrosis. Haematoxylin and eosin stain. Right, mixed histology. Haematoxylin and eosin stain.

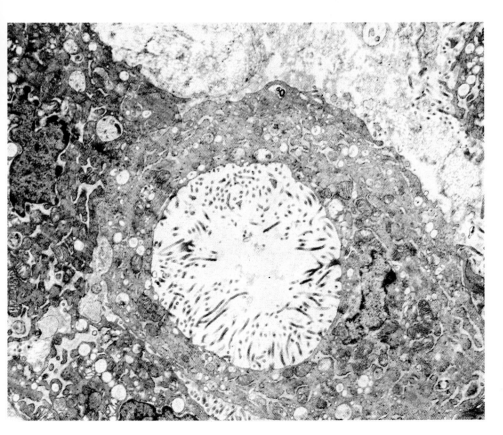

Fig. 3.89 Pleural tumour. Electron microscopy of mesothelioma of the epithelial cell type characterized by long, slender microvilli.

Malignant deposits

Malignant deposits from primary tumours elsewhere in the body may be found in the pleura (Fig. 3.91).

MEDIASTINAL TUMOURS AND CYSTS

It is convenient and of help in diagnosis to group these according to the site where they most commonly occur.

Anterior mediastinum

Thymic tumours

Thymoma is the commonest tumour in the anterior mediastinum; nearly all occur just in front of the base of the heart. The majority are solid but about five to ten percent are cystic. They arise from the epithelial elements of the thymus but there is often an admixture of lymphocytes. In the past, four types have been recognized: lymphocyte-predominant; epithelial; mixed epithelial and lymphocytic; and spindle cell. More recently, separation into cortical, medullary and mixed types

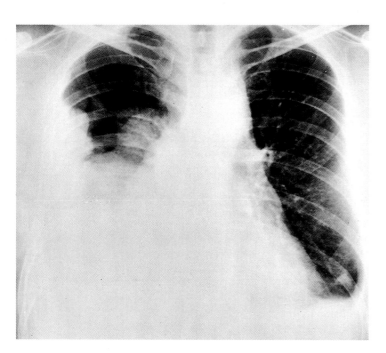

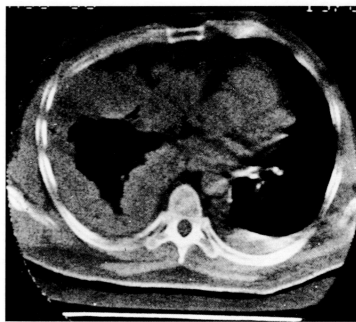

Fig. 3.90 Pleural tumour. Left, nodulated mass along the lateral chest wall and mediastinum and the right base. Appearances are of a pleural tumour. A small left pleural effusion is also present — malignant mesothelioma. Right, CT scan confirms that there is extensive pleural involvement on the right extending through medially behind the heart to the left side where there is a pleural effusion.

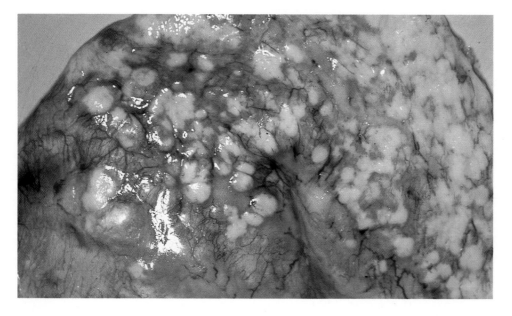

Fig. 3.91 Pleural metastases. Multiple discrete deposits of a metastatic carcinoma.

has been advocated, but it is debatable whether any histological classification is of prognostic significance. Factors such as encapsulation or invasive activity are much more important in this respect. Most thymomas are benign but some spread locally and into the pleura, where they may seed, causing widespread pleural deposits. Areas of necrosis and calcification are often present, the calcification frequently being sufficiently extensive to be visible on a plain chest radiograph.

Approximately half of patients with a thymic tumour have myasthenia gravis and one-fifth of patients with myasthenia have a thymic tumour. As the thymus lies in the midline, thymic tumours may be difficult to identify on frontal chest radiographs where they are hidden by the shadows cast by the spine and other mediastinal structures. When sufficiently large they usually bulge on both sides of the mediastinal shadow. Computed tomography is of particular value in the demonstration of these tumours, especially in patients with myasthenia in whom only small tumours may be present (Fig. 3.92). A rare (six percent) association with thymoma is hypogammaglobulinaemia. Even more rare is anaemia due to erythroid

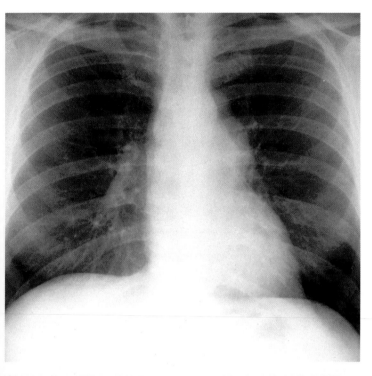

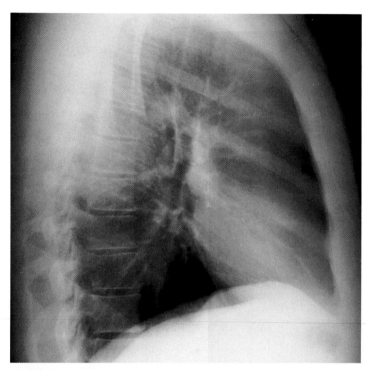

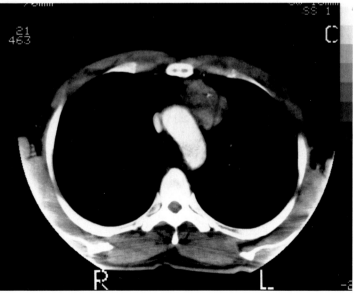

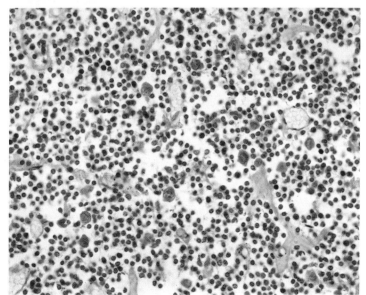

Fig. 3.92 Thymoma in a patient with myasthenia gravis. A lobulated mass is seen in the anterior mediastinum in front of the aortic arch and left hilum. Top left, frontal radiograph. Top right, lateral radiograph. Bottom left, CT scan. A speck of calcification is seen within the lesion. Bottom right, histology showing scanty, single, atypical thymic epithelial cells and a background of reactive lymphocytes. In other thyomas epithelial cells predominate and lymphocytes are scanty but these differing histological patterns have no prognostic significance.

hypoplasia. Occasionally a fatty element of the thymus forms a large thymolipoma in which there is a capsule of thymic tissue surrounding a central tumour of fat; such tumours may become very large. Carcinoid tumours also arise in the thymus, usually in men. They tend to be more aggressive than those that arise in the lungs. Thymic carcinoids may cause Cushing's syndrome or be one component of Wermer's multiple endocrine adenoma syndrome.

Germ cell tumours

These tumours are derived from germ cells in the anterior mediastinum and may become very large. If benign, the lesion is usually cystic — a dermoid cyst — and may contain cholesterol and sebaceous debris, with teeth, bone and calcification within the wall. They are teratomas, often containing ectodermal, mesodermal and endodermal derivatives. About thirty percent of mediastinal germ cell tumours are malignant.

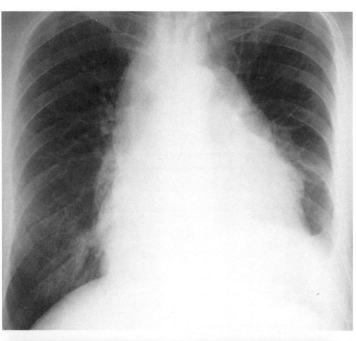
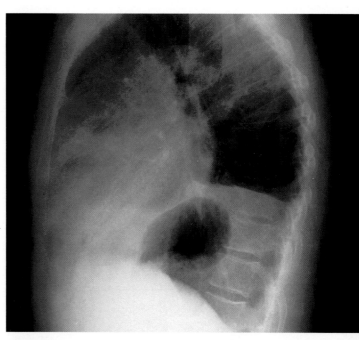
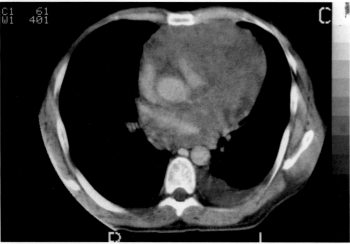
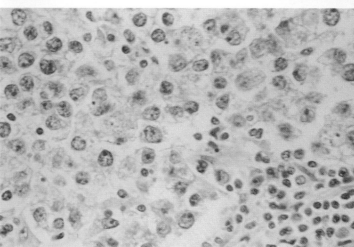

Fig. 3.93 Germ cell tumour of the mediastinum. Top left and top right, radiographs show a large irregular mediastinal mass and a left pleural effusion. The dome of the diaphragm is elevated due to phrenic paralysis. Bottom left, the CT scan at the level of the right pulmonary artery confirms the large mediastinal mass due to an infiltrating tumour surrounding the ascending aorta, pulmonary trunk and the right pulmonary artery. These last two are severely compressed and distorted. The left pleural effusion is evident. Bottom right, histology showing a sheet of polygonal cells with large vesicular nuclei and prominent nucleoli and a group of reactive lymphocytes (bottom right). The appearances are identical to those of testicular seminoma and ovarian dysgerminoma. Other mediastinal germ cell tumours are teratomatous and may be benign (e.g. dermoid cyst) or malignant.

Malignant germ cell tumours may become very large and occupy a large part of the anterior mediastinum. Some have a cell structure identical to seminoma of the testis or dysgerminoma of the ovary. Other malignant varieties consist of extra-embryonic tissue such as yolk sac or chorion. They occur mainly in young men (Fig. 3.93).

Infection of the cystic variety is a serious and not infrequent complication, possibly leading to rupture of the cyst into an airway when the contents, including hair, may be coughed up. Abscesses, fistulae and pulmonary collapse are also complications of infection. The tumours are frequently quite large, often larger than thymic tumours, and are seen at the same site in the anterior mediastinum at the base of the heart. They more frequently bulge to one side of the mediastinum than to both sides. On the chest radiograph they appear as clearly defined smooth round or oval masses when benign and lobulated when malignant (see Chapter 2) (Fig. 3.94). The low density cholesterol and debris within the cyst can be detected radiographically, particularly by CT.

Retrosternal goitre

In a great majority of patients with a mediastinal thyroid there is a direct connection with a palpable thyroid swelling in the neck. The majority extend from the lower pole of the thyroid into the anterior mediastinum in front of the trachea, but the remainder extend from the posterior aspect of the thyroid behind the trachea and the head and neck vessels. Rarely they extend into the posterior part of the mediastinum below the level of the aortic arch and occasionally they are found as low as the pericardium in the anterior mediastinum. Histologically, mediastinal goitre is usually of the nodular colloid variety.

Radiologically, the mass is clearly defined, smooth or slightly lobulated and of uniform density, though calcification may be identified, particularly on CT (Fig. 3.95). The mass frequently displaces and compresses the trachea either from in front or from one side (see Chapter 2). When posterior to the trachea, the goitre displaces the trachea forwards and the oesophagus to one side and posteriorly. Radioactive isotope studies may show the lesion and confirm the diagnosis but frequently retrosternal

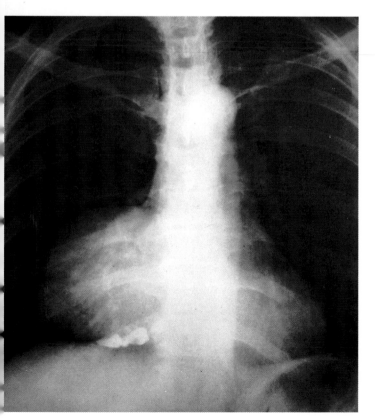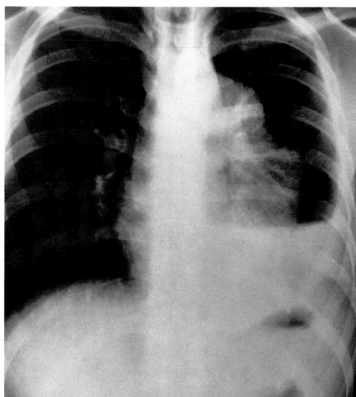

Fig. 3.94 <u>Dermoid cyst</u>. Left, a frontal radiograph showing a cyst with teeth in its lower part. Right, another patient with a left sided dermoid cyst which has become infected causing increase in size of the cyst and a left pleural effusion. A post aspiration pneumothorax is present.

goitres are non-functioning and do not take up the isotope. Patients with retrosternal goitre are usually asymptomatic but may have cough, respiratory embarrassment, stridor and hoarseness due to recurrent laryngeal paralysis. The onset of symptoms may be acute due to a sudden haemorrhage into the goitre causing acute compression of the trachea.

Superior mediastinum

Retrosternal thyroid and lymphadenopathy have already been discussed above. Bronchogenic cysts and aortic aneurysms are covered in the following section.

Middle and posterior mediastinum
Lymphadenopathy

The mediastinum contains an abundance of lymph-nodes in all divisions but mainly concentrated around the major bronchi and the trachea. Evaluation of enlarged lymph-nodes is mainly radiological. At the hilum, lymphadenopathy is probably just as well detected by conventional tomography as by CT but there is no doubt that in the mediastinum CT is the examination of choice.

The causes of lymphadenopathy in the mediastinum are the same as elsewhere in the body.

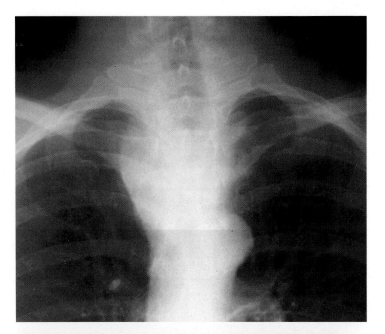

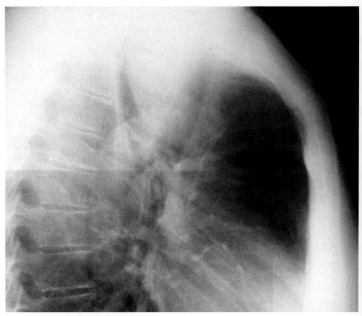

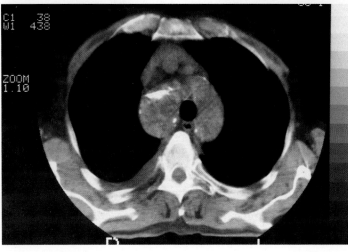

Fig. 3.95 Intrathoracic goitre, Top, frontal and lateral radiographs showing a goitre lying behind and to the right of the trachea which is displaced forwards and to the left at the thoracic inlet. It extends down as far as the level of the arch of the aorta. Bottom, CT scan of a different patient with a partially calcified intrathoracic goitre on the right of the trachea opposite the top of the aortic arch.

Infection

Enlargement of nodes in the hilum and mediastinum may occur in any acute lung infection such as pneumonia, but is seldom detected except in children. Some chronic infections such as those in cystic fibrosis cause enlargement of hilar and mediastinal lymph-nodes. As part of the generalized infection, enlarged mediastinal nodes are rarely seen on the chest radiograph in infectious mononucleosis (glandular fever) but are often very large in the much rarer infection, bubonic plague (*Yersinia* (*Pasteurella*) *pestis* infection). The commonest infection in which enlarged hilar and mediastinal nodes are found is tuberculosis (Fig. 3.96), often part of a primary complex. Histoplasmosis and coccidioidomycosis, prevalent in the United States of America, are other infections which are associated with mediastinal lymphadenopathy. Central irregular calcification of nodes occurs in tuberculosis, histoplasmosis and coccidioidomycosis when healing occurs.

Benign hyperplasia (Castleman's disease)

Castleman described an unusual form of lymphadenopathy in which a solitary mass is present — usually mediastinal or hilar. The mass consists of widely scattered lymphoid follicles in which there is penetration by many capillaries.

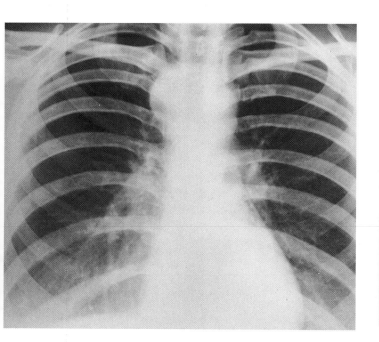

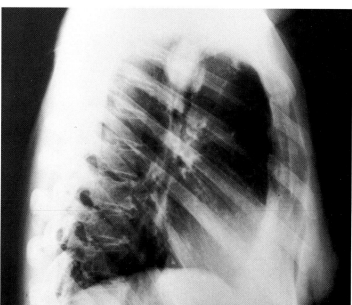

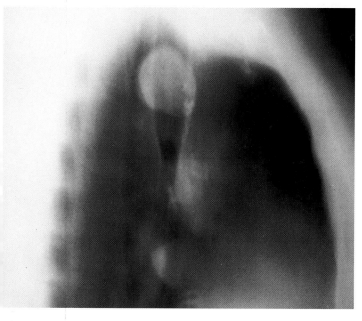

Fig. 3.96 Tuberculous lymphadenopathy. A smooth swelling is seen on the right side of the superior mediastinum due to enlarged paratracheal lymph nodes. Top left, frontal radiograph. Top right, lateral radiograph. Bottom, lateral tomogram.

Sarcoidosis
Sarcoidosis is characterized by hilar and mediastinal node enlargement.

Silicosis
In silicosis, hilar and mediastinal lymph-node enlargement is often seen. The nodes are not greatly enlarged and may calcify; the calcification occurring in the rims of the nodes, so-called egg shell calcification, similar to that seen in sarcoidosis.

Lymphoma and leukaemia
Hodgkin's disease is the most frequent lymphoma to affect the mediastinal lymph-nodes and is one of the commonest causes of mediastinal lymph-node involvement. About seventy percent

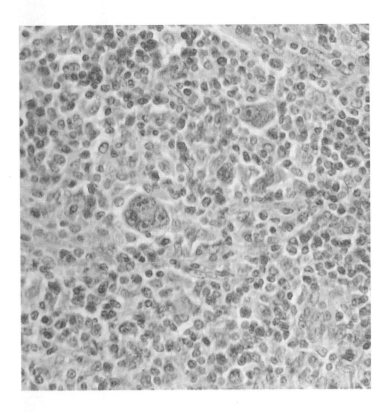

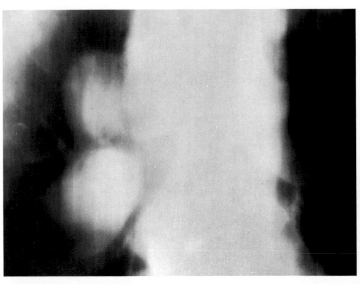

Fig. 3.97 Hodgkin's disease. Right, large lymph nodes are seen on a tomogram in the right hilum, in the right tracheobronchial angle, around the carina and to the right of the trachea. The left hilum is normal though there are some enlarged nodes on the left side of the superior mediastinum. Note the asymmetrical distribution. Left, histology showing two Reed–Sternberg cells and a heavy infiltrate of eosinophils.

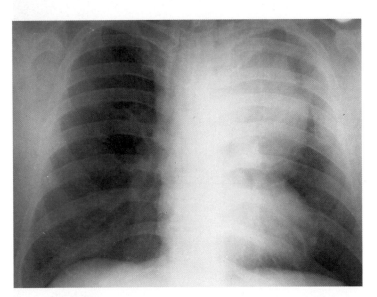

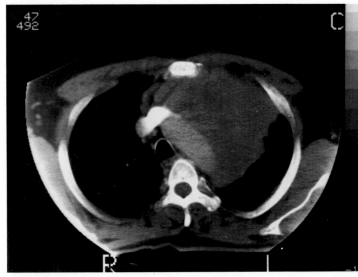

Fig. 3.98 Hodgkin's disease. A large left sided superior mediastinal mass is present. The computed tomogram shows this extending across the mid line in front of the superior vena cava and lying to the left and in front of the aortic arch which is displaced to the right with the trachea. Biopsy revealed the mass to be due to Hodgkin's disease. Left, frontal radiograph. Right, CT scan (contrast enhanced).

of patients with Hodgkin's disease have mediastinal lymphadenopathy (Fig. 3.97). Hilar nodes may also be involved, often asymmetrically, unlike sarcoidosis in which symmetrical enlargement of the hilar nodes is usual, though not invariable. The massive enlargement of nodes may cause compression of adjacent structures, particularly the superior vena cava with consequent obstruction. Involvement of the thymus and the lymph-nodes in the internal mammary chains in the superior mediastinum may give rise to retrosternal masses (Fig. 3.98). This occurs most frequently in young patients with nodular sclerosing Hodgkin's disease which is often associated with cervical node involvement. Calcification of lymph-nodes in Hodgkin's lymphoma occurs only after treatment with cytotoxic drugs or radiotherapy.

Non-Hodgkin's lymphoma may affect any of the mediastinal nodes and the diagnosis can only be made by histological examination. Frequently the intrathoracic manifestations are only one part of a widespread generalized disease. A higher incidence of non-Hodgkin's lymphoma, particularly the histiocytic variety, occurs in patients who are immunosuppressed or immunodeficient.

In leukaemia, mediastinal and hilar node enlargement is the commonest intrathoracic feature and is more common in lymphocytic leukaemia than in the myeloid type. Pleural effusion and pulmonary infiltration are less frequent than node enlargement.

Metastatic carcinoma

One of the commonest causes of mediastinal lymph-node enlargement is metastatic involvement by carcinoma of the bronchus (Fig. 3.99). Sometimes the primary lesion is difficult to detect in the lungs or is very small, in spite of a large

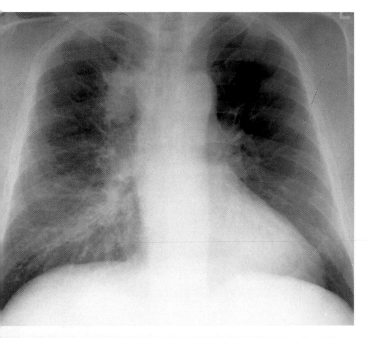

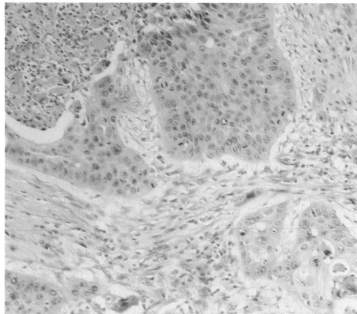

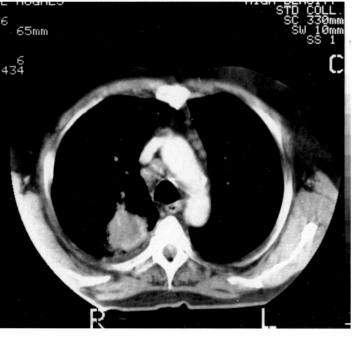

Fig. 3.99 Squamous cell carcinoma in the right upper lobe. The frontal chest radiograph shows a lesion in the lung together with some enlargement of nodes at the right hilum and in the right paratracheal region. Bottom left, CT scan shows nodes greater than 1cm between the trachea and SVC and also to the left of the aortic arch confirming extensive mediastinal lymph node involvement. The histology shows infiltrating cords of stratified epithelium with a high mitotic index. Keratinization is evident bottom right and necrosis top left.

mediastinal mass. Symptoms arise from pressure on surrounding structures, cough and dyspnoea being the commonest. Facial swelling due to obstruction of the superior vena cava and phrenic nerve and recurrent laryngeal nerve paralysis also occur. The detection of hilar and mediastinal nodes for staging of carcinoma of the bronchus is of utmost importance in management and treatment.

Normal lymph-nodes are usually less than 1cm in diameter. In the staging of carcinoma of the bronchus, mediastinal lymph-nodes less than 1cm in diameter on computer tomography show histological evidence of involvement in five to six per-cent, but if over 1.5cm in diameter invasion by tumour is found in ninety-four to ninety-seven percent. A node over 1cm in diameter should therefore be regarded with a high degree of suspicion.

Metastases from other primary malignant tumours include carcinoma of the upper intestinal tract, oesophagus, prostate, breast and kidney.

Bronchogenic cysts

The majority of bronchogenic cysts are situated adjacent to the trachea or one of the major airways (Fig. 3.100). They

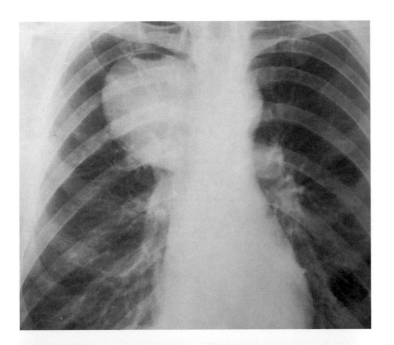

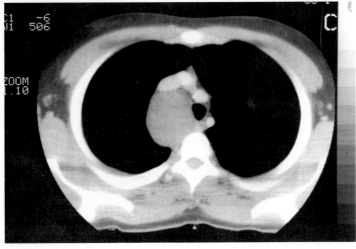

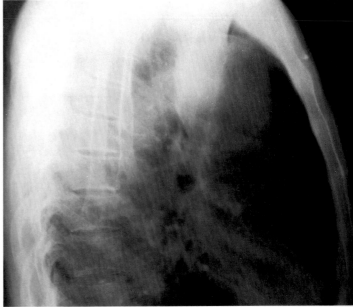

Fig. 3.100 Bronchogenic cyst. Top, frontal and lateral radiographs showing a clearly defined opacity on the right side of the trachea. A small air fluid level is seen in the upper part of the cyst due to a very small communication with the bronchial tree. Bottom, CT scan of a similar lesion without a fluid level. The density of the contents is that of fluid.

are lined with bronchial mucosa and contain liquid mucoid material. Rarely there is a communication with the bronchial tree when a fluid level may be seen within the cyst on the chest radiograph. They rarely produce symptoms but may become infected in which case they can increase rapidly in size and produce symptoms not only of the infection but also from compression of adjacent airways. Radiologically they are seen as smooth, clearly defined masses adjacent to the trachea or main bronchi. Widening of the carina may be present — similar to that seen due to an enlarged left atrium with which a cyst may be confused.

Pleuropericardial cysts

These cysts almost never cause symptoms, nor do they become infected; they are usually chance findings on routine chest radiographs. They may communicate with the pericardium and are thought to be developmental in origin arising from errors in differentiation of coelomic cavities. Radiologically the cysts are smooth, round or oval, projecting from the heart border (Fig. 3.101). Sometimes they are found in the interlobar fissures and on the diaphragm and they are frequently found in the anterior cardiophrenic angle. They commonly range from 3–8 cm in diameter and contain clear fluid.

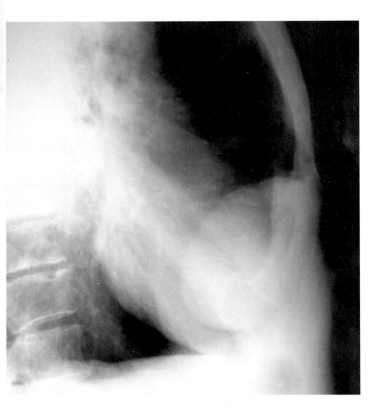

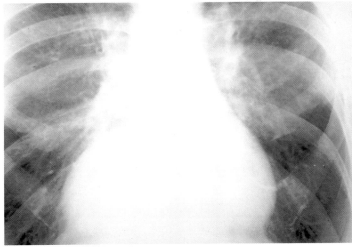

Fig. 3.101 Pleuropericardial cyst. Radiographs showing smooth clearly defined mass on the right border of the heart anteriorly. On the lateral view it is seen to be separate from the diaphragm.

Lipoma

The mediastinum normally contains a variable amount of fat, and lipomas may occur in any part. They often reach a great size before symptoms occur and are frequently a chance finding on the radiograph (see Chapter 2). They may be seen on plain radiographs to be of low density, but this is readily demonstrable by CT (Fig. 3.102). Generalized lipomatosis of the mediastinum may occur as a complication of steroid therapy. Lipomas in the lower mediastinum should be differentiated from diaphragmatic hernias, which may contain omental fat. Bowel may be demonstrated within such a hernia either by CT or a barium meal and follow-through examination.

Duplication cysts of the oesophagus

Similar to bronchogenic cysts but rarer, duplication cysts of the oesophagus are developmental cysts arising from the foregut. They occur adjacent to the oesophagus, with which they may communicate (Fig. 3.103), and are lined with oesophageal, gastric or even intestinal mucosa.

Neuroenteric cysts

These cysts are also developmental cysts of the foregut and arise as a result of failure of complete separation of the endoderm from the notochordal plate during embryonic development; they are lined by both gastrointestinal and neural elements. They occur in the posterior mediastinum adjacent to the oesophagus and are usually connected to the meninges by a stalk, and occasionally to the gastrointestinal tract below the diaphragm. Communication to the gastrointestinal tract may be patent and allow the cyst to be filled by gas. Because of the connection with the meninges defects in the upper dorsal vertebrae are frequently present (Fig. 3.104). Very rarely this communication is patent and cerebrospinal fluid from the subarachnoid space may be found in the cyst. The communication can be demonstrated by myelography.

Aneurysms of the aorta

Aneurysms of the aorta may be saccular or fusiform. They result from atherosclerosis, trauma, cystic medial necrosis and syphillis. Mycotic aneurysms of the aorta are very rare.

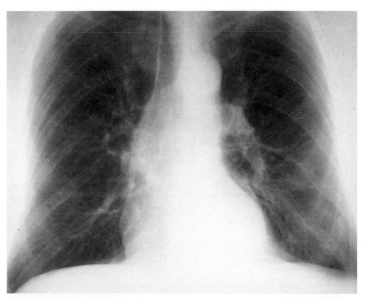

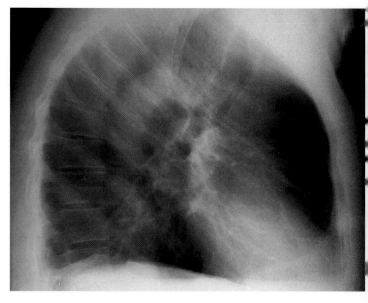

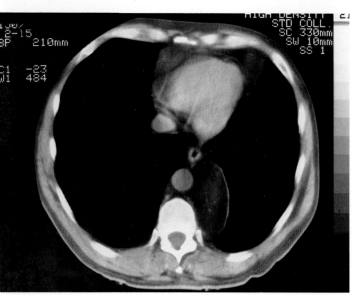

Fig. 3.102 Lipoma of the mediastinum. Top left and top right, chest radiographs showing a lower density smooth opacity behind the heart on the left side of the mediastinum. Bottom, CT scan showing that the tumour is fatty and is lying to the left of the descending aorta and spine.

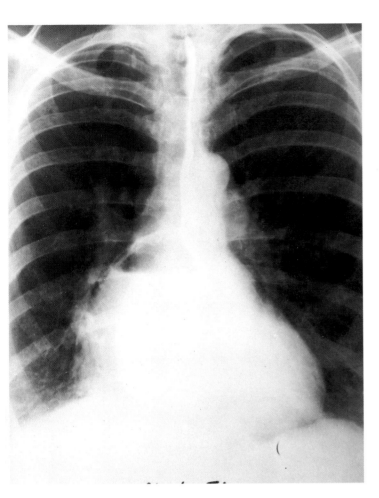
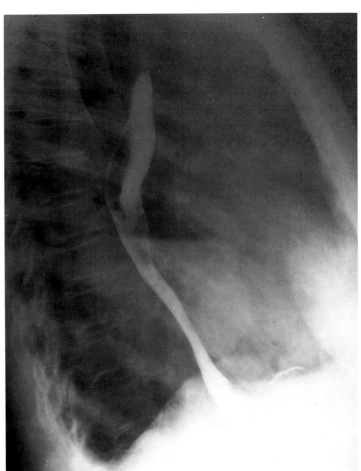

Fig. 3.103 Foregut cyst. Left and right, chest radiographs with barium in the oesophagus. The cyst which has an air fluid level is seen lying close to the right side of the lower half of the oesophagus. Though the cyst did not fill with barium there was a communication with the oesophagus which permitted air to get into it.

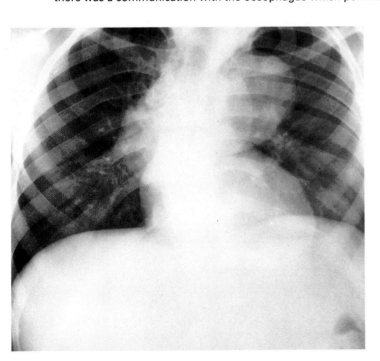
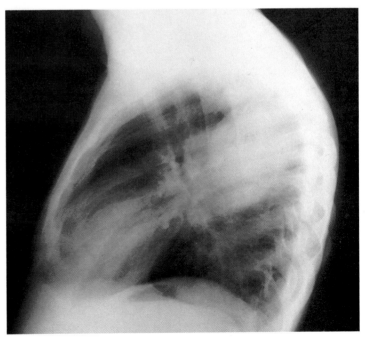

Fig. 3.104 Neuroenteric cyst. Left and right, radiographs of a child with a lobulated cyst on either side and in front of the spine which has numerous defects causing a mid dorsal kyphosis.

Tumours of the oesophagus

Carcinoma is the commonest tumour of the oesophagus. The presenting symptom is dysphagia. The tumour is usually of insufficient size to be visible on a plain chest radiograph when discovered, though it may cause deformity of the posterior mediastinal line, or the azygo-oesophageal recess. On computed tomography the mass can be identified and its limits in the mediastinum defined. Carcinoma of the oesophagus has a poor prognosis.

Benign tumours are rare, but when they occur they may be very large before discovery and dysphagia is a late symptom. Leiomyoma is the commonest type, but fibromas, lipomas and hamartomas occur. Projection of the tumour into the lumen of the oesophagus may cause a large polypoid mass to be formed within the lumen on a relatively small stalk. The mass is frequently detected on a plain chest radiograph to the right and in front of the descending aorta and filling the azygo-oesophageal recess (Fig. 3.105).

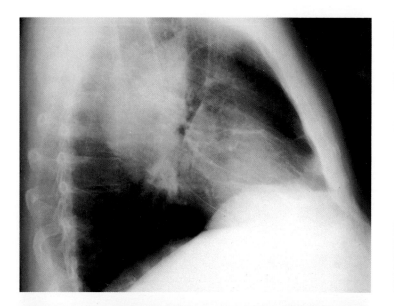

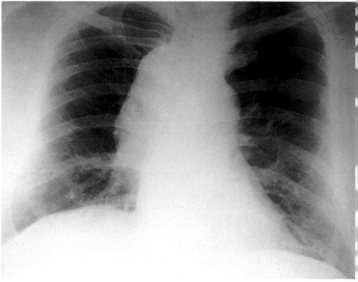

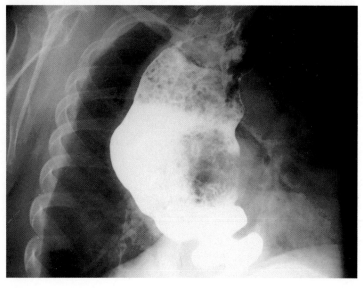

Fig. 3.105 Leiomyoma of the oesophagus. Top, chest radiographs. A large mass is seen in the posterior mediastinum displacing the trachea and main bronchi forward. The mass bulges to the right from the level of the thoracic inlet to the level of the right dome of the diaphragm. Bottom, a barium swallow shows a very large intraluminal filling defect in the oesophagus. The tumour was a pedunculated leiomyoma. The patient had very few symptoms with only occasional dysphagia.

Neurogenic tumours

Neurogenic tumours are second only to retrosternal thyroid in frequency amongst the mediastinal masses. They include neurofibroma (from the nerve sheath), neurilemmoma (from the sheath of Schwann), ganglioneuroma (from the sympathetic ganglia), ganglioneuroblatoma (usually malignant), neuroblastoma (highly malignant) and paraganglioma (phaechromocytoma and chemodectoma).

Neurofibromas and neurilemmomas mostly arise from the intercostal nerves and rarely from the vagus and phrenic nerves. Neurofibromas may be part of generalized neurofibromatosis (Von Recklinghausen's disease). They appear as smooth, round or oval masses usually in the angle between the vertebral body and the posterior ends of the ribs (Fig. 3.106). The ribs may show evidence of pressure, splaying and erosion caused by the tumour and there may be widening of the intervertebral foramen, particularly if there is an intraspinal component of the tumour.

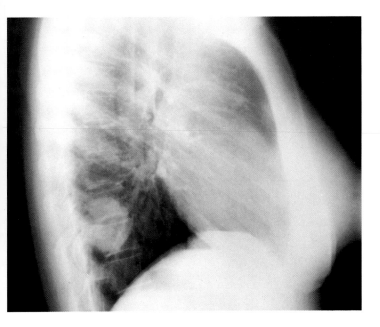

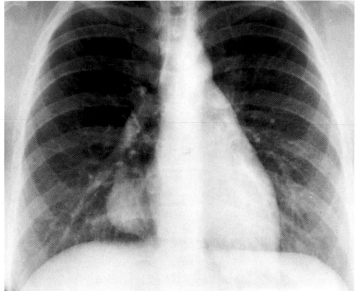

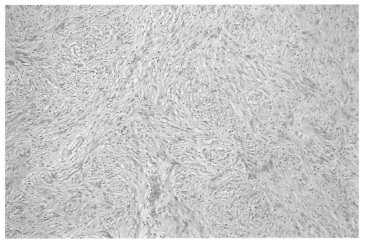

Fig. 3.106 Paravertebral neurofibroma. Top, chest radiographs. A smooth round mass is seen in the right paravertebral gutter. There is slight splaying of the adjacent ribs but no other evidence of bone erosion and no widening of the intervertebral foramen. Bottom, histology showing interweaving bundles of spindle cells.

These tumours also occur along the course of the intercostal nerves in the chest wall and appear then as extrapleural masses on the chest radiograph. Ganglioneuromas occur along the sympathetic chain, as do neuroblastomas; they lie more ante- riorly than neurofibromas, along the side of the vertebral body, and appear as paravertebral smooth oval masses with a broad mediastinal base on chest radiographs. Punctate calcifi- cation may be visible within the tumours.

Meningocoele
This rare cause of a posterior mediastinal mass is due to herniation of the meninges through the intervertebral foramen. The appearances of the lesion are similar to neurofibroma with a smooth round paravertebral mass at any level of the thoracic spine. The lesion often causes enlargement of the intervertebral foramen and may be associated with a thoracic scoliosis. Vertebral and rib anomalies are often associated and the lesion may occur in association with generalized neurofibromatosis. It is important to recognize this lesion before a surgical resection of what is thought to be a neurofibroma is undertaken. The meningocoele may be demonstrated by myelography or by computed tomography, when a connection with the spinal canal can be seen.

Tumours of the spine
Tumours of the spine and posterior aspects of the ribs may invade the posterior mediastinum and paravertebral gutter (Fig. 3.107).

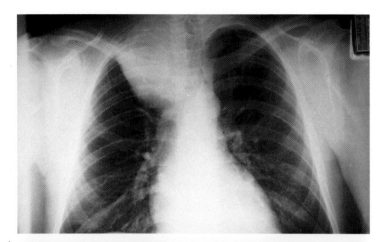

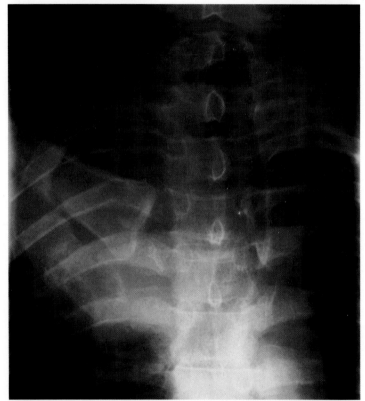

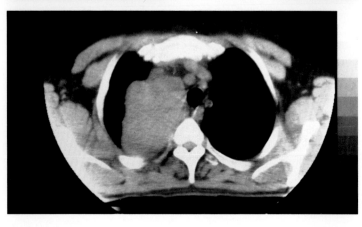

Fig. 3.107 Giant cell tumour of rib. The chest radiograph, top, shows a mass on the right side of the upper mediastinum displacing the trachea slightly to the left. Middle, a film of the dorsal spine shows destruction of the medial end of the right second rib. The head and neck of the rib are missing. They should lie just below the transverse process of the vertebra which is intact. Bottom, CT scan showing the mass extending forwards on the right side of the mediastinum.

Index